Pelvic Dysfunction in Men

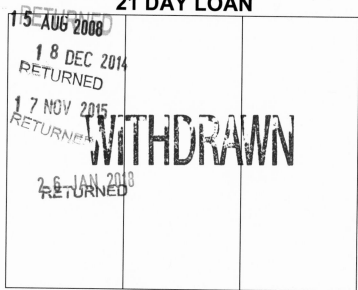

Pelvic Dysfunction in Men
Diagnosis and Treatment of Male Incontinence and Erectile Dysfunction

A textbook for physiotherapists,
nurses and doctors

Professor Grace Dorey, PhD, FCSP
Professor of Physiotherapy, University of the West of England, Bristol
Senior Research Fellow, University of Aberdeen
Extended Scope Practitioner, North Devon District NHST Hospital, Barnstaple
Consultant Physiotherapist, The Somerset Nuffield Hospital, Taunton

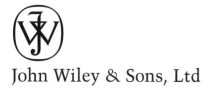

John Wiley & Sons, Ltd

Copyright © 2006   John Wiley & Sons Ltd
The Atrium, Southern Gate, Chichester,
West Sussex PO19 8SQ, England
Telephone (+44) 1243 779777

Email (for orders and customer service enquiries): cs-books@wiley.co.uk
Visit our Home Page on www.wiley.com

Other Wiley Editorial Offices
John Wiley & Sons Inc., 111 River Street, Hoboken, NJ 07030, USA
Jossey-Bass, 989 Market Street, San Francisco, CA 94103-1741, USA
Wiley-VCH Verlag GmbH, Boschstr. 12, D-69469 Weinheim, Germany
John Wiley & Sons Australia Ltd, 42 McDougall Street, Milton, Queensland 4064, Australia
John Wiley & Sons (Asia) Pte Ltd, 2 Clementi Loop #02-01, Jin Xing Distripark, Singapore
129809
John Wiley & Sons Canada Ltd, 6045 Freemont Blvd, Mississauga, ONT L5R

Wiley also publishes its books in a variety of electronic formats. Some content that appears
in print may not be available in electronic books.

Library of Congress Cataloging-in-Publication Data
Dorey, Grace.
    Pelvic dysfunction in men : diagnosis and treatment of male incontinence and erectile
dysfunction : a textbook for physiotherapists, nurses and doctors / Grace Dorey.
      p. ; cm.
    Includes bibliographical references and index.
    ISBN-13: 978-0-470-02836-0 (alk. paper)
    ISBN-10: 0-470-02836-X (alk. paper)
    1. Urinary incontinence–Diagnosis.   2. Urinary incontinence–Treatment.   3. Impotence–
Diagnosis.   4. Impotence–Treatment.
    [DNLM: 1. Urinary Incontinence–diagnosis.   2. Impotence–diagnosis.   3. Impotence–
therapy.   4. Urinary Incontinence–therapy. WJ 146 D695p 2006]   I. Title.
    RC921.I5D67 2006
    616.6′2–dc22
                    2006004909

A catalogue record for this book is available from the British Library
ISBN – 13   978-0-470-02836-0
ISBN – 10   0-470-02836-X

Typeset by SNP Best-set Typesetter Ltd., Hong Kong
Printed and bound in Great Britain by TJ International Ltd, Padstow, Cornwall

Dedication

To my friend and physiotherapy colleague Claire Oldroyd, who referred my first male urology patient to me in 1996.

To Dr John Oldroyd, my first male urology patient, a delightful man who inspired me to research the subject in greater depth.

Contents

List of Figures

6. URINARY INCONTINENCE

8. PATIENT ASSESSMENT

9. CONSERVATIVE TREATMENT

10. LITERATURE REVIEW OF TREATMENT BEFORE AND AFTER PROSTATECTOMY

11. TREATMENT OF POST-PROSTATECTOMY PATIENTS

13. FAECAL INCONTINENCE

14. MALE SEXUAL DYSFUNCTION

15. TREATMENT OF MALE SEXUAL DYSFUNCTION

List of Tables

Preface

This textbook follows my first textbook published in 2001 entitled *Conservative Treatment of Male Urinary Incontinence and Erectile Dysfunction*. It contains seven new chapters and existing chapters have been extensively updated. It is written primarily for those specialist continence physiotherapists who are unsure of the treatment for male patients with lower urinary tract symptoms. It will be a useful reference tool for urology nurses, continence specialist nurses and continence advisors; and those medical students, student nurses and physiotherapy students suddenly finding themselves on a urology placement. It will provide a greater knowledge of conservative treatment in this speciality for urologists and GPs. Where possible, the information is based on the current literature, even though this remains sparse in some areas. The avid reader and the questioning research student may find the references provide further, fascinating and more in-depth reading.

There is a new chapter concerning the history of the male pelvic floor. Our understanding of the male pelvic floor has evolved over more than two thousand years. Gradually medical science has sought to dispel ancient myths and untruths.

Background details concerning the prevalence of male lower urinary tract symptoms, the anatomy and physiology of the pelvic floor and the physiology of the continence mechanism are provided in order to understand the dysfunction that can occur. A new chapter entitled 'Nervous control of lower urinary tract function' provides current thinking and new diagrams concerning bladder and sphincter reflexes.

The different prostatic conditions are covered in detail, plus the range of standardised medical and surgical investigations and treatments. The classification of male urinary incontinence has been restructured in line with the International Continence Society standardisation of terminology. The subjective and objective physiotherapy assessment is covered chronologically, to enable the clinician to conduct a meaningful investigation and arrive at a logical diagnosis.

Recommended therapeutic options are provided for each type of incontinence, with a range of patient advice added for completeness. Treatment outcomes, which may vary considerably, are discussed. Following the treatment chapter, there are case studies, which provide question and answer sessions for the student to check their knowledge base.

There are two new chapters covering the conservative treatment of men who have experienced prostate surgery. The first of these chapters reviews the evidence from randomised controlled trials for post-prostatectomy patients. The second chapter provides details of treatment regimes for these men.

There is a novel chapter detailing treatment regimes for men with faecal incontinence.

There are two new chapters covering the conservative treatment for men with sexual dysfunction. The first of these chapters explains the range of sexual dysfunction in men. The second chapter provides details of treatment regimes for these men based on current evidence from literature reviews.

The Appendix includes an updated male continence assessment form.

In the Glossary at the end of the book, definitions have been added to explain the medical jargon, as some readers may not have a medical background, while others may lack knowledge of some of the obscure urology terminology.

I hope you will find this book interesting, informative and a useful reference source. Enjoy your studies.

Indeed, it is the book that I would have welcomed before embarking on my MSc. It contains information which I have gathered, analysed and compiled over the last nine years.

Acknowledgements

I would like to acknowledge the help of some very special people. I am indebted to Debbie Rigby, Stephanie Knight, Professor Michael Craggs, Mr Raj Persad, Jane Dixon, Tracy James and Jeannie Smith for their contribution, wisdom and guidance. Importantly, I would like to thank my son, Martin, and daughter, Claire, for the support and encouragement they have given me in my chosen field and my daughter, Claire, for her accurate anatomical illustrations.

Grace Dorey

Illustrator

Claire Dorey, BA

1 History of the Male Pelvic Floor

Key points

- In 400 BC, it was believed that air flowed into the penis to effect an erection.
- In 1519, it was first known that blood flow was responsible for penile erection.
- In AD 47, the electric eel was used to gain an anal contraction.
- In 1930, pelvic floor muscle exercises were first taught.
- In 1901, the pelvic floor muscles were first linked to penile erection.

INTRODUCTION

Our understanding of the male pelvic floor has evolved over more than two thousand years. Gradually medical science has sought to dispel ancient myths and untruths. Anatomists have held erroneous theories for hundreds of years based on the hypotheses of great men such as Hippocrates in 400 BC and later Leonardo da Vinci in the sixteenth century (Chadwick & Mann 1987; Van Driel et al. 1994). The male pelvic floor was not mentioned in the first anatomy book by Quain or in the first edition of Gray's *Anatomy* (Quain 1828; Gray 1858). Since then, anatomists have documented the anatomy and physiology of the male urogenital diaphragm, termed the pelvic floor in subsequent editions (Figure 1.1).

PHYSIOTHERAPY DEVELOPMENT

Physiotherapy treatment has evolved over the last 110 years in the UK. It commenced in 1894 when 'The Society of Trained Masseuses' was founded by four nurses from The London Hospital. In 1919, this society amalgamated with 'The Institute of Massage and Remedial Exercises' established in Manchester and in 1920 the Royal Charter was granted and the two bodies became 'The Chartered Society of Massage and Medical Gymnastics'. In 1944, the Society in the UK adopted its present name as the 'Chartered Society of Physiotherapy'. In 1964, Vidler stated that 'You needed a good educational background to train as a physiotherapist, but when qualified it is wit and observation that give you the ability to judge the effect of your treatment and report on it or discuss it

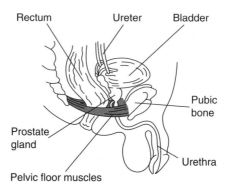

Figure 1.1. Male pelvic floor muscles (Reproduced by permission of NEEN Mobilis Healthcare Group. *Source*: Dorey, 2004b)

with the doctor' (Vidler 1964). It was not until 1977 that Chartered Physiotherapists became autonomous clinicians in the UK, with the ability to take self-referrals, assess, diagnose and treat without a medical referral.

In 1964, Rule 2 of the Code of Conduct stated that registered physiotherapists should confine themselves to the recognised field of physiotherapy (Gardiner 1964). Physiotherapy was extremely protective of its core skills of massage, exercises and electrotherapy (added in 1929). At this stage, it lacked the foresight and courage to develop new skills in other areas. Physiotherapists were generalists and expected to undertake all types of physiotherapy treatment. Gradually, physiotherapy skills have expanded to cover many specialist areas, such as continence. Now, physiotherapists confine themselves to areas in which they have had training and in which they are competent. In 1992, the profession became an all-graduate entry profession in the UK.

Physiotherapy treatment for female incontinence has gradually evolved over the last 66 years, whilst physiotherapy treatment for male incontinence has evolved more recently. Up till 1997, nurses in the UK dominated the management of male continence problems. Since then, physiotherapists have been active in teaching pelvic floor exercises and providing patients with relevant advice (Dorey 2000).

ASSESSMENT OF THE MALE PELVIC FLOOR

Before 1996, there was no recognised method of assessing the strength of the pelvic floor muscles in men. In 1996, Wyndaele and Van Eetvelde found that digital anal assessment of the pelvic floor muscles, grading from 0 (nil) to 5 (strong), was a reliable method of testing pelvic floor muscle strength in men.

Dorey and Swinkels (2003) found anal manometry to be a reliable outcome measurement for pelvic floor muscle strength. Following a randomised controlled trial of pelvic floor muscles for men with erectile dysfunction, Dorey (2004a) argued the need for another digital anal grade for men, grade 6 (very strong).

PELVIC FLOOR EXERCISES

The earliest reference to muscle relaxation and muscle strengthening was found in the Ebers Papyrus (c. 3000–1534 BCE) (Ebbell 1937). The earliest mention of pelvic floor exercises was found in a book dedicated to 'medical gymnastics and massage' (Arvedson 1930). Swedish Medical Gymnastics were used by physiotherapists in 1938 to strengthen the pelvic floor muscles in women (Prosser 1938). Strong, resisted concentric muscle activity of the hip adductors was used to work the pelvic floor muscles. Two gymnasts stood either side of the patient positioned in supported supine lying whilst resistance was applied to hip adduction. Eccentric work of the pelvic floor was effected when the gymnasts drew the legs out whilst the patient continued to work the hip adductors strongly (Prosser 1938).

Dr Arnold Kegel has always been considered the pioneer of pelvic floor muscle exercises for women, even though Swedish Gymnastics preceded his work (Kegel 1948). In 1948, he proposed postnatal pelvic floor muscle exercises and, to his credit, pelvic floor muscles are still termed 'Kegels' in America. Gardiner (1959) demonstrated four exercises (Figure 1.2) which worked the muscles of the pelvic floor, but all these exercises worked the hip adductors and buttocks as well as the pelvic floor muscles.

POSTURE

In 1938, Prosser wrote that the human body in the standing position is in a state of unsteady equilibrium, as its centre of gravity is a long way from its base. In 2001, Sapsford et al. reported that muscle stability of the body was achieved by the action of the diaphragm working in conjunction with the pelvic floor muscles, and the transverse abdominal muscles working in conjunction with the multifidus muscles of the spine.

DETRUSOR UNDERACTIVITY

In 1930, Dr Arvedson recommended catheter treatment and gymnastic treatment for paralysis of the bladder. Gymnastic treatment consisted of bladder shaking, perineal shaking, back hacking and gentle sacral beating to stimulate

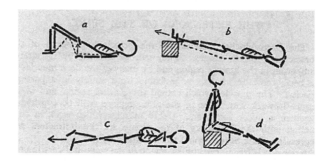

Key

a. Crook lying (with pelvis lifted); brace buttocks, press knees together, and pull up between legs.

b. Leg lift lying (heels supported and legs crossed); hip raising and adduction with pelvic floor contraction.

c. Side lying (legs bent); leg stretching and adduction with pelvic floor contraction.

d. Inclined long sitting (ankles crossed); brace buttocks, press knees together and contract pelvic floor.

Figure 1.2. Early pelvic floor exercises (*Source*: Gardiner, 1995)

contraction of the bladder; and crook-half-lying, knee closing and parting with pelvis lifting to strengthen and improve the tone of the muscles of the pelvic floor (Arvedson 1930).

DETRUSOR OVERACTIVITY

In 1960, Muellner first described bladder training for child bed-wetters with detrusor overactivity. Children were encouraged to hold on for longer periods of time. Burgio et al. (1989) first used biofeedback and bladder training for men with detrusor overactivity. Patients were encouraged to stand or sit

quietly during the urge and relax the abdominal muscles and contract the urinary sphincter muscles until the urge had diminished. They were then advised to walk at normal pace to the toilet.

In 1977, Mahony et al. suggested that a pelvic floor contraction during urgency would inhibit a detrusor contraction via the perineal-pudendal reflex.

NOCTURNAL ENURESIS

In 1930, Dr Ardveson advised the first treatment regime for nocturnal enuresis consisting of banning evening drinks, telling the patient not to wet the bed, cold sponging to the perineum morning and evening, waking him once during the night and gymnastic treatment. In 2002, Nijman et al. treated this condition by using a positive attitude, pelvic floor muscle exercises, a reward system for children following dry nights, desmopressin medication, and not drinking for 2 hours before bedtime.

POST-PROSTATECTOMY INCONTINENCE

The first radical prostatectomies were performed in India by Freyer in 1901 and in the UK by Young in 1904 (Garrison 1917). Sir Eardley Holland coined the term 'stress incontinence' to describe exertional incontinence in women (Millin & Read 1948). In 1957, post-prostatectomy patients were prone to chest complications and thrombosis and were therefore allowed to get out of bed early (Cash 1957). Physiotherapists performed leg massage and leg exercises.

The first estimate of urinary incontinence following transurethral resection of prostate in 1983 found an incidence of 1.5 % after surgery (Habib & Luck 1983). In 1966, the incidence increased to 32.5 % at three months after surgery, possibly due to subjective reporting (Emberton et al. 1996).

The first estimate of urinary incontinence following radical prostatectomy in 1984 found an incidence of 87 %, six months after surgery (Rudy et al. 1984). In 1997, the incidence reduced to 36 % at the same assessment time owing to improved surgery using nerve-sparing techniques (Donnellan et al. 1997).

In 1959, Gardiner taught patients with stress incontinence to brace the pelvic floor muscles before any activity which raised the intra-abdominal pressure, such as coughing, sneezing, laughing or lifting heavy weights. This bracing was termed 'The Knack' in 1996 by Miller et al. in recognition of the fact that the skill needed to be learned.

In 1976, Sotiropoulos et al. used electrical stimulation for men with post-prostatectomy incontinence with a 45 % success rate. In 1989, Burgio et al.

treated post-prostatectomy stress incontinence with biofeedback and 51 pelvic floor muscle contractions a day with some success. In 1994, Opsomer et al. undertook the first randomised controlled trial of pelvic floor exercises plus anal electrical stimulation versus no treatment for post-prostatectomy incontinence. Results showed no between-group significant difference, but both groups were taught pelvic floor muscle exercises. In 2001, Sueppel et al. were the first to demonstrate that pre-prostatectomy pelvic floor muscle exercises reduced incontinence after radical prostatectomy.

Moore et al. (2000) produced the first Cochrane Review of randomised controlled trials using pelvic floor exercises for post-prostatectomy incontinence and concluded that it was not possible to reliably identify or rule out a useful effect. Van Kampen et al. (2000) demonstrated the significant effectiveness of pelvic floor exercises for men after radical prostatectomy. Various methods have been employed to strengthen the pelvic floor muscles. Wisinski et al. (2001) used a rectal weight to strengthen up the pelvic floor muscles following post radical prostatectomy incontinence in a case study of one subject.

POST-MICTURITION DRIBBLE

In 1970, Vereecken and Verduyn, using a pressure sensor and electromyography, noticed an increase in urethral pressure and a visible contraction of the bulbocavernosus muscle expelling the last drops of urine at the end of micturition. In 1977, Stephenson and Farrar, using videocystography during mid-stream stopping, demonstrated that men with post-micturition dribble failed to milk urine back into the bladder during contraction of the external urethral sphincter. They suggested that men apply manual compression to the bulbar urethra in the perineum after micturition. Paterson et al. (1997) were the first to show in a randomised controlled trial that pelvic floor exercises or bulbar urethral massage was significantly effective for post-micturition dribble. Dorey et al. (2004b) demonstrated that pelvic floor muscle exercises were significantly effective in curing post-micturition dribble and superseded bulbar urethral massage for this condition.

CONSTIPATION

In 1899, Bruce treated constipation with a 'habitual pill of aloes and strychnine until they regain the muscular tone which they have lost'. In 1903, Elliman treated constipation with 'massage of the belly daily' using Elliman's embrocation for 20 minutes or rolling a 6 lb metal ball over the abdomen for 5 to 10 minutes every morning. Also, alternate douching of the abdomen with hot and cold water was used to excite bowel activity. In 1938, Prosser treated

chronic constipation with abdominal massage and colon frictions to increase the flow of blood to the gut and stimulate peristalsis.

FAECAL INCONTINENCE

Historically, prolapsed anus and faecal incontinence were treated with electric shock treatment to gain a contraction of the anal sphincter. The first use of electrotherapy was recorded in AD 47 by Scribonius Largus, who described the use of the electric eel for prolapsed ani (Gadsby 1998). In 1601, William Gilbert, discovered materials termed 'electra' and coined the term 'electricity' (Gadsby 1998). Johann Krueger, professor of philosophy and medicine, published the first medical electricity textbook entitled *Thoughts about Electricity* in 1744 (Gadsby 1998). Faradism was used in 1898 by Dommer in Germany for bed-wetting, applying one electrode over the urethra and one over the anus (Stainbrook 1948). In 1920, a physician named Eberhart used high-frequency current for a variety of rectal diseases. He used a mild spark for treating prolapsed rectum to cause an immediate contraction, and used a spark and then a rectal tube for relieving the itching of pruritis ani. Men with paralysis of the anal sphincter were given rectal applications and spark to the spine. Gardiner (1959), a physiotherapist, performed anal faradic stimulation using an anal electrode so that patients could feel an anal contraction with the instruction 'Draw up the back passage'. Since then, faradism has been replaced by electrical stimulation, which is a more comfortable form of treatment.

ERECTILE DYSFUNCTION

In 400 BC, Hippocrates believed that erections were generated by air and 'vital spirits' flowing into the penis. He also believed that the testes were connected to the penis by a pulley system of erectile cords which facilitated erection, as damage to these cords profoundly affected penile erection. Leonardo da Vinci (1452–1519) found that men executed by hanging developed a reflex erection and that dissection of the penis showed it to be full of blood, not air (Friedman 2003). After dissecting more than 30 corpses, Leonardo believed that semen came from the brain, along the spinal cord to the penile tube.

In 1901, Poirier and Charpy first reported that contractions of the ischiocavernosus and bulbocavernosus muscles were necessary to attain a full erection. In 1909, Gray's *Anatomy* published a lithograph of the male urogenital diaphragm labelling the ischiocavernosus muscle 'erector penis' and the bulbocavernosus muscle 'ejaculator urine'. In 1973, Beckett et al. found that there was increased pelvic floor muscle activity in the stallion during coitus. In 1983, Karacan et al. investigated the activity of the ischiocavernosus and bulbocavernosus muscles during nocturnal erections using electromyography. They concluded that these muscles played a role in the erection in man. Lavoisier et al. (1986) demonstrated an increase in intracavernous pressure in the penis during contractions of the ischiocavernosus and bulbocavernosus muscles.

For the last ten years, the term 'impotence' has been considered offensive and has gradually been replaced with the term 'erectile dysfunction' and, in 2004, the International Society for Sexual and Impotence Research (ISSIR) eventually changed its name to the International Society for Sexual Medicine (ISSM).

Kawanishi et al. (2000) devised a novel method of giving resisted exercises to the ischiocavernosus muscle. They strapped a spring balance to the coronal groove of the penis to measure the maximum strength of this muscle and found that the potent men were significantly stronger than impotent men. In 1993, Claes and Baert compared pelvic floor exercises with deep dorsal vein suturing in men with erectile dysfunction and obtained similar results in both groups. In 1999, Colpi et al. using electromyography found that the pelvic floor muscles were significantly stronger in sexually active men than men with erectile dysfunction. Two randomised controlled trials have demonstrated significant improvement in erectile function with pelvic floor exercises. In 2002, Sommer et al. found pelvic floor exercises to be superior to Viagra and in 2004, Dorey et al. found that pelvic floor exercises were significantly more effective than lifestyle changes for men with erectile dysfunction (Dorey et al. 2004a).

CONCLUSION

Our conception of the male pelvic floor has altered considerably over time. Early erroneous assumptions have been dispelled with diagnostic techniques such as anatomical dissection, electromyography, videocystography, manometry, digital anal assessment, and surgery. Recent good research has added considerably to our fund of knowledge.

2 Lower Urinary Tract Symptoms

Key points

- Moderate to severe lower urinary tract symptoms occur in 29–51 % of men in the UK aged 50 years and over.
- Lower urinary tract symptoms in men can be divided into storage symptoms, voiding symptoms, post-micturition symptoms, and genital and lower urinary tract pain.
- Storage symptoms include urgency, urge urinary incontinence, nocturia, frequency and stress urinary incontinence.

MALE LOWER URINARY TRACT SYMPTOMS

Lower urinary tract symptoms are defined from the man's perspective, who is usually, but not necessarily, a patient within the healthcare system (Abrams et al. 2002). In elderly men, whilst many of the symptoms are caused by benign prostatic hyperplasia, up to one-third of the symptoms have other causes, such as detrusor overactivity and detrusor underactivity (Kortmann et al. 1999). Lower urinary tract problems contribute to social and psychological problems which may severely affect quality of life. Lower urinary tract symptoms can be divided into storage symptoms, voiding symptoms, post-micturition symptoms, and genital and lower urinary tract pain (Abrams et al. 2002).

STORAGE SYMPTOMS

Storage symptoms are experienced during the storage phase of the bladder, and include daytime frequency and nocturia (Abrams et al. 2002). Other storage symptoms are urgency, urge urinary incontinence, stress urinary incontinence, nocturnal enuresis and continuous urinary incontinence (Table 2.1).

VOIDING SYMPTOMS

Voiding symptoms are experienced during the voiding phase (Abrams et al. 2002). Voiding symptoms include slow stream, intermittent stream, hesitancy, straining and terminal dribble (Table 2.1).

Table 2.1. Lower urinary tract symptoms in men (*Source*: Abrams et al. 2002)

Storage symptoms	Voiding symptoms	Post-micturition symptoms
Daytime frequency	Slow stream	Feeling of incomplete
Nocturia	Intermittent stream	emptying
Urgency	Hesitancy	Post-micturition dribble
Urge urinary incontinence	Straining	
Stress urinary incontinence	Terminal dribble	
Nocturnal enuresis		
Continuous urinary		
incontinence		

POST-MICTURITION SYMPTOMS

Post-micturition symptoms are experienced immediately after micturition (Abrams et al. 2002). Post-micturition symptoms include a feeling of incomplete emptying and post-micturition dribble.

GENITAL AND LOWER URINARY TRACT PAIN

Pain, discomfort and pressure are part of a spectrum of abnormal sensations felt by the individual (Abrams et al. 2002). Pain produces the greatest impact on the patient and may be related to bladder filling or voiding, may be felt after micturition, or be continuous (Chapter 7).

MALE QUESTIONNAIRES

International Prostate Symptom Score

Urologists and general practitioners use prostate symptom scores in order to assess the severity of prostatic symptoms and determine the need for surgery for the obstruction. Various unvalidated prostate symptom scores have been used previously, but these were replaced in 1991 by the International Prostate Symptom Score (I-PSS) validated by the International Continence Society (ICS). In order to assess the severity of lower urinary tract symptoms, patients report whether they have suffered from the following symptoms within the last month:

Incomplete emptying
Frequency
Intermittency
Urgency

Weak stream
Straining
Nocturia

Each question is scored 0–5 giving a possible total of 35:

0 = not at all
1 = less than 1 time in 5
2 = less than half the time
4 = more than half the time
5 = almost always

Patients are also asked to rate their quality of life due to their urinary symptoms from the following seven categories:

1. Delighted
2. Pleased
3. Mostly satisfied
4. Mixed, about equally satisfied and dissatisfied
5. Mostly dissatisfied
6. Unhappy
7. Terrible

There is controversy as to the need for a prostate symptom score. Vestey and Hinchcliffe (1998) in a prospective study of 126 consecutive men with lower urinary tract symptoms compared the I-PSS to a 7-day bladder diary. They found that 64 % of men overestimated their frequency and 47 % overestimated their nocturia on the I-PSS questionnaires. Half the scores revealed nocturnal polyuria (>33 % urinary output during bedtime hours) with 11 % of men producing greater than 50 % of their output at night. There was no correlation between the I-PSS and post-void residual volumes for incomplete bladder emptying, and no correlation between the I-PSS and maximum flow rates for patients with a weak stream. They concluded that the bladder diary, in combination with uroflowmetry and post-void residuals, answered the I-PSS questions more objectively and in more detail than the I-PSS questionnaire. In addition, the bladder diary provided important information on nocturnal output, co-morbidity and social habits. They recommended the routine use of bladder diaries for the assessment of male lower urinary tract symptoms.

ICS*male* questionnaire

The ICS*male* questionnaire was compiled because some urinary symptoms are unrelated to prostatic outflow obstruction (Donovan et al. 1996). This provides a more accurate way to assess male urinary symptoms. The ICS*male* questionnaire contains questions on 20 urinary symptoms, 19 of which have an additional question to ascertain the degree of bother that they cause. It is easy for the patient to complete. The questions on frequency and nocturia demonstrate reasonable agreement with bladder diaries but there is a poor relationship between questions assessing stream and the results of uroflowmetry. It was shown to have good internal consistency and good test–retest reliability. It was considered a breakthrough for assessing the severity of lower urinary tract symptoms.

Quality of life

Quality of life has been linked to the World Health Organization (WHO) definition of health, which was defined as a state of physical, emotional and social well-being, and not just the absence of disease or infirmity (World Health Organization, 1978). The quality of life is subjective. The I-PSS has only one question concerning quality of life. The International Continence Society Quality of Life questionnaire (ICSQoL) assesses men's quality of life due to lower urinary tract symptoms (Donovan et al. 1997).

PREVALENCE OF LOWER URINARY TRACT SYMPTOMS

Moderate to severe lower urinary tract symptoms (LUTS) are relatively common. They occurred in 29–51 % of a sample of 1,088 men aged 50 years and over in the UK (Trueman et al. 1999) (see Table 2.2). However, the researchers only assessed urinary symptoms and ignored pain when they used the International Prostate Symptom Score (I-PSS) as the method of assessment. Only half the men with moderate to severe symptoms had sought medical attention. The main reasons given for not seeking a consultation were 'symptoms may get worse', 'fear of cancer', 'interruption to daily activities' and 'embarrassment'.

Moderate to severe lower urinary tract symptoms occur in about 25 % to 30 % of men aged 50 years and over who have not had surgery and the preva-

Table 2.2. Age-specific prevalence of men with moderate to severe LUTS (Reproduced with permission of Blackwell Publishing Ltd, *Source*: Trueman et al., 1999)

Age group (years)	Sample, n	Symptomatic, n (%)
All (50–92)	1088	452 (41)
50–60	14	4 (29)
61–70	330	124 (38)
71–80	598	247 (41)
>80	146	75 (51)

LUTS = lower urinary tract symptoms.

lence increases with age (Chute et al. 1993; Garraway et al. 1991; Hunter et al. 1996). The symptoms of urgency, frequency and nocturia were found to be present in 50 % of men aged 62–90 years in the USA who had not undergone surgery (Milne et al. 1972). The symptoms of bladder outlet obstruction, most commonly due to benign prostatic hyperplasia, were reported to affect 1 in 3 men over the age of 50 years in the UK (Garraway et al. 1991).

SUMMARY

Lower urinary tract symptoms can be divided into storage symptoms, voiding symptoms, post-micturition symptoms, and genital and lower urinary tract pain. The ICS*male* questionnaire coupled with the ICS*QoL* questionnaire provides a more accurate way to assess male lower tract symptoms than the I-PSS.

3 Anatomy and Physiology of the Lower Urinary Tract

Key points

- The lower urinary tract consists of the urinary bladder and the urethra.
- The prostate gland surrounds the prostatic segment of the proximal urethra.
- The pelvic floor muscles are divided into a superficial layer and a deep layer.
- The male pelvic floor muscles have a number of different functions.

MALE LOWER URINARY TRACT

The lower urinary tract consists of the urinary bladder and the urethra. The proximal urethra is surrounded by the prostate gland above and the external urethral sphincter and pelvic floor muscles below.

URINARY BLADDER

The urinary bladder is a hollow organ located in the true pelvis (Figure 3.1). It consists of four layers: the outer protective adventitia, the detrusor muscle, the vascular submucosa and the urothelium. The complex meshwork of smooth muscle bundles of the detrusor muscle are interspersed with collagenous supporting tissue (Gray 1992).

MALE URETHRA

The male urethra is between 18 and 20 cm long and extends from the bladder neck through the prostate and the penile shaft to its meatus at the glans penis as shown in Figure 3.2. It is divided into the proximal (sphincteric) and the distal (conduit) segments. The proximal urethra is further divided into the prostatic urethra which extends approximately 3 cm through the prostate, and the membranous urethra, which is approximately 3.5 cm long and lies just below the prostate where it pierces the pelvic floor muscles (Gray 1992). Midway between the base and the apex

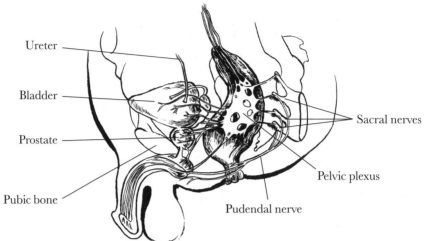

Figure 3.1. Male pelvic viscera (Reproduced by permission of John Wiley & Sons, 2001. *Source*: Dorey 2001b)

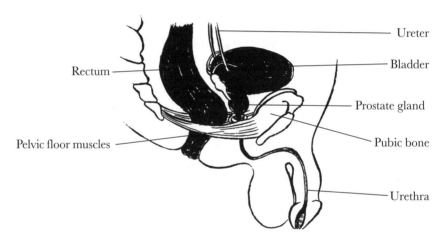

Figure 3.2. Male lower urinary tract (Reproduced by permission of John Wiley & Sons, 2001. *Source*: Dorey, 2001b)

of the prostate gland, the prostatic urethra angulates ventrally at about 35 degrees (Sant & Long 1994). The proximal urethra contains smooth muscle bundles and the specialised skeletal muscle fibres of the horse-shoe-shaped external urethral sphincter (rhabdosphincter) and an inner urothelium which is lined by transitional epithelium and abundant secretory cells.

PROSTATE GLAND

The prostate gland is a small, walnut-shaped, fibromuscular gland with ducts sited at the base of the bladder surrounding the prostatic urethra as shown in Figure 3.3. The young adult prostate is about $4 \times 3 \times 2$ cm in size and weighs about 20 g but increases with age (Neal 1997).

The prostate gland produces fluid which provides one of the constituents of semen. Seminal fluid contains nutrients, such as zinc (antibacterial factor) and citrate (sperm transport) enabling sperm motility and mobility (Sant & Long 1994). Prostate-specific antigen (PSA), a protein secreted by the prostate gland, may be found in the blood stream. At ejaculation the prostate acts as a pump. The smooth muscle of the bladder neck contracts to prevent urine escaping and semen entering the bladder during ejaculation. The prostate gland may gradually enlarge with age in the presence of androgens, especially dihydrotestosterone, causing benign prostatic hyperplasia (BPH). When microscopic changes become macroscopic, symptoms of urethral obstruction may develop (Neal 1997) (Table 3.1).

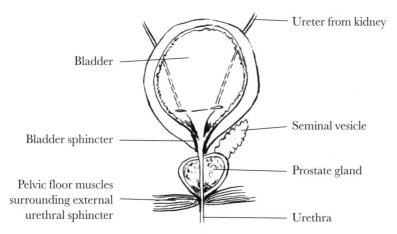

Figure 3.3. Prostate gland (Reproduced by permission of John Wiley & Sons. *Source*: Dorey, 2001b)

Table 3.1. The prevalence of clinical BPH and symptoms with ageing (Reproduced by permission of Blackwell Publishing Ltd. *Source*: Neal 1997)

Age (years)	Microscopic (%)	Gross (%)	Severe symptoms (%)
35–44	8	2	0
45–54	23	8	0
55–64	42	21	2–5
65–74	71	35	8–15
75–84	82	44	15–20
>85	88	53	20–30

PELVIC FLOOR MUSCLES

In the male the pelvic floor muscles extend from the anterior to the posterior of the bony pelvis, forming a diaphragm covering the pelvic outlet which supports the urethrovesical system and rectum. The puborectalis muscle forms a sling from the pubic bone round the rectum at the anorectal junction. The pelvic floor muscles are divided into a deep and a superficial layer.

Gosling et al. (1981) reported that the pelvic floor muscles were made up of about two-thirds type 1, slow-twitch, aerobic oxidative fibres which were continuously tonic to support the pelvic viscera. The periurethral striated muscle is a mixture of fast and slow twitch muscle fibres that raise urethral closure pressure during periods of increased intra-abdominal pressure or by voluntary control (DeLancey 1994).

DEEP PELVIC FLOOR MUSCLES

The deep layer consists of the external urethral sphincter, puborectalis, pubococcygeus, iliococcygeus, and ischiococcygeus muscles. The deep pelvic floor muscles are shown in Figures 3.4 and 3.5.

Levator ani

The levator ani consists of the pubococcygeus muscle and the iliococcygeus muscle. The pubococcygeus and iliococcygeus muscles together with the ischiococcygeus muscle form a muscular diaphragm which supports the pelvic viscera and opposes the downward thrust caused by an increase in intra-abdominal pressure.

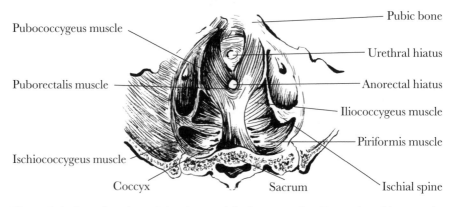

Figure 3.4. Superior view of the deep pelvic floor muscles (Reproduced by permission of John Wiley & Sons. *Source*: Dorey, 2001b)

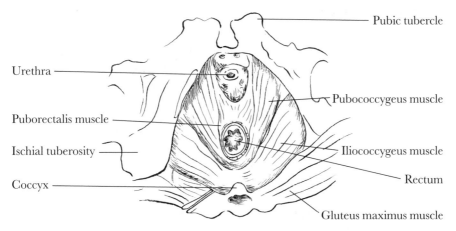

Pubic tubercle

Urethra

Pubococcygeus muscle

Puborectalis muscle

Ischial tuberosity

Iliococcygeus muscle

Coccyx

Rectum

Gluteus maximus muscle

Figure 3.5. Inferior view of the deep pelvic floor muscles (Reproduced by permission of John Wiley & Sons. *Source*: Dorey, 2001b)

Pubococcygeus muscle

The pubococcygeus muscle arises from the back of the pubic bone and the anterior part of the obturator fascia and inserts into a fibro-muscular layer between the anal canal and the coccyx. The pubococcygeus muscle draws the coccyx forward after defaecation.

Iliococcygeus muscle

The iliococcygeus muscle arises from the ischial spine and from the tendinous arch (arcus tendineus) of the pelvic fascia and is attached to the coccyx and the median raphe. The pubococcygeus muscle draws the coccyx forward after defaecation.

Ischiococcygeus muscle

The ischiococcygeus muscle arises from the pelvic surface of the ischial spine and is inserted into the side of the coccyx and lower sacrum. It is responsible for pulling the coccyx forward after defaecation.

Puborectalis muscle

The puborectalis muscle arises from the pelvic surface of the pubic bone, blends with the levator ani and is inserted into the muscle from the other side posterior to the rectum at the anorectal flexure. It can be considered part of the pubococcygeus muscle. It helps to maintain faecal continence by maintaining the anorectal angle.

External urethral sphincter

The intrinsic striated muscle of the external urethral sphincter mechanism in the urethra is called the rhabdosphincter (Dixon & Gosling 1994). It surrounds the membranous urethra and lies deep to the urogenital diaphragm. It comprises slow-twitch fibres of small diameter without muscle spindles and is postulated to receive triple innervation from the sympathetic, parasympathetic and somatic nervous systems (Gray 1998). The superficial muscle fibres arise from the transverse perineal ligament and surrounding fascia and insert into the perineal body. The deep fibres form a continuous circular formation round the membranous urethra. The muscles from both sides together form a sphincter compressing the membranous urethra and assisting in the maintenance of urinary continence. They are relaxed during micturition and at the end of micturition, together with the bulbocavernosus muscles, they eject the last few drops of urine.

Gosling et al. (1981) reported the presence of only slow-twitch fibres in the rhabdosphincter. However, in a study using histochemical and electron microscopic techniques, Light et al. (1997) suggested that the rhabdosphincter consisted of two-thirds slow-twitch fibres and one-third fast-twitch fibres, which enabled the sphincter to maintain urethral closure at rest and during physical activity.

Male continence mechanism

The continence mechanism in men consists of the continuous smooth muscular structure of the bladder base, the bladder neck and the proximal urethra supplemented by the striated muscle fibres of the horseshoe-shaped rhabdosphincter (Elbadawi 1995). It was Elbadawi who led thinking away from the previous concept of a separate internal and external sphincter describing instead a 'continuous' continence mechanism. The proportion of striated muscle cells in the rhabdosphincter decreases with age from approximately 79 % in infants to 35 % in an 83-year-old man (Strasser et al. 1997).

SUPERFICIAL PELVIC FLOOR MUSCLES

The superficial layer consists of the external anal sphincter and transverse perineal, bulbocavernosus and ischiocavernosus muscles (Figure 3.6).

Anal sphincter

The anal sphincter consists of elliptical-shaped muscle fibres each side of the anal canal attached to the tip of the coccyx posteriorly and inserted into the perineal body anteriorly. Inferiorly it blends with the skin surrounding the anus and superiorly it forms a complete sphincter and blends with the puborectalis muscle. It is in a normal state of tonic contraction but can provide greater occlusion of the anal aperture when needing to contain faeces and flatus.

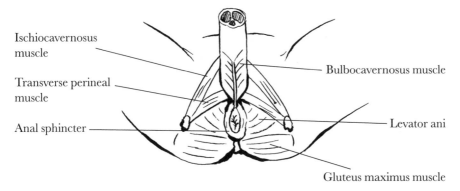

Ischiocavernosus muscle

Transverse perineal muscle

Anal sphincter

Bulbocavernosus muscle

Levator ani

Gluteus maximus muscle

Figure 3.6. Male superficial pelvic floor muscles (Reproduced by permission of John Wiley & Sons. *Source*: Dorey, 2001b)

Bulbocavernosus muscle

The bulbocavernosus muscle, also called the bulbospongiosus muscle, arises from the median raphe and the perineal body. The middle fibres encircle the bulb and corpus spongiosum penis. The bulbocavernosus muscle empties the urethra at the end of micturition. The middle fibres assist in erection of the corpus spongiosum penis by compressing the erectile tissue of the bulb. The anterior fibres spread out over the side of the corpus cavernosum and are attached to the fascia covering the dorsal vessels of the penis and contribute to erection by compressing the deep dorsal vein of the penis. The bulbocavernosus muscle empties the bulbar canal of the urethra. The fibres are relaxed during voiding and come into action to arrest micturition. Rhythmic contractions of the bulbocavernosus muscle propel the semen down the urethra resulting in ejaculation.

Ischiocavernosus muscle

The ischiocavernosus muscle arises from the inner surface of the ischial tuberosity and pubic ramus and inserts into an aponeurosis into the sides and under surface of the crus penis. Contractions of the ischiocavernosus muscles produce an increase in the intracavernous pressure and influence penile rigidity (Chapter 15).

Cremaster muscle

This muscle originates from the middle of the inguinal ligament where its fibres are continuous with the internal oblique muscle and occasionally with the transversus muscle. It passes anterior and lateral to the spermatic cord through the inguinal ring to insert into the cremasteric fascia surrounding the testis. The muscle fibres ascend along the medial and posterior surface of the cord and are inserted into the pubic tubercle and crest of the pubis and front of the rectus abdominis sheath. The cremaster muscle pulls the testis towards the inguinal ring during a strong contraction of the pelvic floor muscles. Stroking the medial side of the thigh evokes a reflex contraction of this muscle (cremasteric reflex). The cremaster muscle is not usually under voluntary control. It is supplied by the genital branch of the genitofemoral nerve (L1 and 2).

PENIS

The penis consists of three cylindrical erectile bodies: dorsally, the two corpora cavernosa communicate with each other for three-quarters of their length and ventrally the corpus spongiosum surrounds the penile portion of the urethra. The proximal end of the corpus spongiosum forms a bulb attached to the urogenital diaphragm and at the distal end expands to form the glans penis (Kirby et al. 1999).

NERVE SUPPLY TO THE URINARY SYSTEM

The autonomic nervous system includes all efferent pathways having ganglionic synapses outside the central nervous system (Levin & Wein 1995). It includes all smooth muscle cells. It is divided into the sympathetic and parasympathetic divisions (Figure 3.7). The sympathetic division supplying the urinary system consists of fibres originating in the thoracic and lumbar regions (T10–L2) of the spinal cord whilst the parasympathetic consists of fibres originating in the cranial and sacral nerves (S2, 3, 4). The function of the sympathetic division is to allow bladder storage. The function of the parasympathetic division is to produce a sustained bladder contraction in response to stimulation of the pelvic nerves.

The normal innervation of the lower urinary tract consists of three systems, which must co-ordinate for normal bladder filling and voiding:

1. *Cholinergic system* controlling the bladder. The cholinergic system refers to those receptors sites in the bladder at which acetylcholine is the neurotransmitter. Cholinergic contractile receptor sites can be blocked by the muscarinic atropine.
2. *Adrenergic system* controlling the bladder and urethra. The adrenergic system refers to those receptor sites at which catecholamine is the neurotransmitter. It includes most postganglionic sympathetic fibres and those fibres to the smooth muscle of the lower urinary tract. Adrenergic receptors are classified either α or β. The α-adrenergic effects cause vasocon-

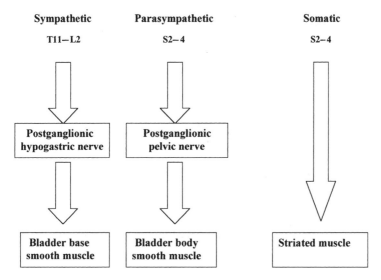

Figure 3.7. Preganglionic and postganglionic neurotransmitters (Reproduced by permission of John Wiley & Sons. *Source*: Dorey, 2001b)

striction and contraction of smooth muscle fibres, whereas β-adrenergic effects cause vasodilation and smooth muscle relaxation.

The bladder is innervated by the second, third and fourth sacral nerves (S2–4). The nerve supply to the external urethral sphincter is an area of debate. Studies in cats suggest that it is innervated by a combination of autonomic nerves via the pelvic plexus and somatic nerves via the pudendal nerve (Elbadawi & Schenk 1974). Studies by Narayan et al. (1995) demonstrated innervation by several branches from the dorsal nerve of the penis after it splits from the pudendal nerve.

3. *Somatic nerves* (pudendal nerves) serving the pelvic floor muscles. The external anal sphincter is supplied by the perineal branch of the fourth sacral nerve and by twigs from the inferior rectal branch (S2, 3) whereas the levator ani, ischiococcygeus and bulbocavernosus are supplied by the perineal branch of the pudendal nerve (S2, 3, 4).

SACRAL DERMATOMES

The dermatome from the second sacral nerve (S2) extends over the lateral aspect of the buttocks and thigh and the posterior aspect of the calf and plantar surface of the heel. The dermatome from the third sacral nerve (S3) covers an area over the upper two-thirds of the medial aspect of the thigh. The dermatome from the fourth sacral nerve (S4) extends over the penis and perineal area (Figure 3.8).

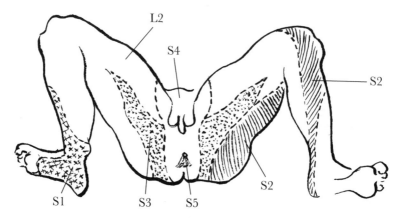

Figure 3.8. Sacral dermatomes (Reproduced by permission of John Wiley & Sons. *Source*: Dorey, 2001b)

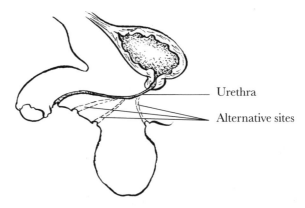

Figure 3.9. Hypospadias (Reproduced by permission of John Wiley & Sons. *Source*: Dorey, 2001b)

CONGENITAL ABNORMALITIES

HYPOSPADIAS

Hypospadias is a congenital abnormality where the urethral meatus opens on the underside (ventral surface) of the penis anywhere along the penis from the meatus to the scrotum (Figure 3.9). It may be associated with chordee where the glans penis bends ventrally and the penis has a ventral angulation. It is usually repaired in the young by surgery.

EPISPADIAS

More rarely encountered, epispadias is a congenital abnormality where the urethral meatus opens at an abnormal position on the upper (dorsal surface) of the penis (Figure 3.10). It is usually repaired in the young by surgery.

URETHRAL VALVES

Occasionally, young boys may be born with urethral valves caused by an abnormal fold of the urethra in the prostatic, membranous or proximal bulbar section (Caldamone 1994). These valves cause reflux of urine, with the danger of hydronephrosis and ultimately renal failure. Early surgical intervention is paramount.

URETERAL VALVES

Occasionally, young boys may be born with malformed and incompetent ureteral valves at the junction of the ureter and bladder. These valves cause reflux of urine, with the danger of hydronephrosis and ultimately renal failure. Early surgical intervention is paramount.

EXSTROPHY OF THE BLADDER

A serious congenital abnormality occurs when the abdominal wall fails to develop and the bladder fails to close leaving the ureters on the surface of the abdomen and the bladder exposed (Caldamone 1994) (Figure 3.11).

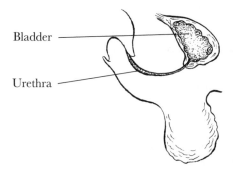

Figure 3.10. Epispadias (Reproduced by permission of John Wiley & Sons. *Source*: Dorey, 2001b)

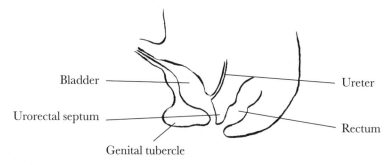

Figure 3.11. Exstrophy of the bladder (Reproduced by permission of John Wiley & Sons. *Source*: Dorey, 2001b)

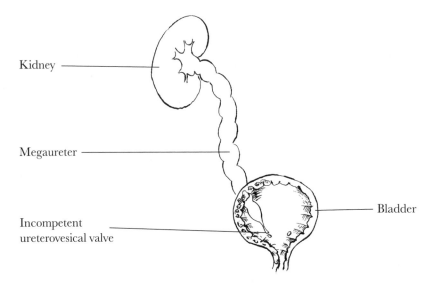

Kidney

Megaureter

Incompetent
ureterovesical valve

Bladder

Figure 3.12. Megaureter (Reproduced by permission of John Wiley & Sons. *Source*:
Dorey, 2001b)

The bladder has to be reconstructed surgically or the ureters diverted through
the abdominal wall using a portion of the ileum to form an ileal conduit.

URETERAL ECTOPIA

An ectopic ureter is a ureter with its insertion directly into the urethra
instead of the trigone area of the bladder. If the insertion level is below
the external urethral sphincter, it may cause continuous incontinence. It is
sometimes associated with duplex ureters. Ureteral ectopia is repaired by
surgery.

PRIMARY OBSTRUCTIVE MEGAURETER

A primary obstructive megaureter is due to a derangement of the ureteral
musculature which impedes the normal peristalsis conveying a bolus of urine
(Caldamone 1994) (Figure 3.12). A developmental arrest of the longitudinal
musculature may lead to a nonperistaltic segment of ureter causing
obstruction.

SECONDARY OBSTRUCTIVE MEGAURETER

An incompetent ureteral valve at the lower end of the ureter as it passes
through the bladder wall may cause secondary reflux and a megaureter.

SUMMARY

The lower urinary tract consists of the urinary bladder and the urethra. The prostate gland surrounds the prostatic segment of the proximal urethra. The pelvic floor muscle can be divided into a deep and a superficial layer. Congenital abnormalities may occur affecting any part of the urinary system.

4 Nervous Control of Lower Urinary Tract Function

Key points

- The continence mechanism in men consists of the bladder base, the bladder neck and the proximal urethra supplemented by the rhabdosphincter.
- Urinary continence relies on an intact urinary system with a competent urethral sphincter and integration of the peripheral nerves, spinal cord, pons and cerebral cortex.
- Neurological integral reflexes control bladder storage and voiding.

INTRODUCTION

The lower urinary tract is innervated by three sets of peripheral nerves: pelvic parasympathetic nerves, lumbar sympathetic nerves and pudendal nerves (Morrison et al. 2005). These nerves contain sensory afferent axons as well as efferent pathways.

URINARY CONTINENCE

Urinary continence relies on three mechanisms: an anatomically intact urinary system; integration of neural modulatory structures in the brain, spinal cord and peripheral nervous system; and a competent urethral sphincter mechanism (Gray 1992; Park et al. 1997). Maintenance of urinary continence is multifactorial and depends on detrusor control and urethral closure function (Bernstein 1997). Passive urethral closure is enhanced by the activity of the rhabdosphincter muscle and the use of the pelvic floor muscles, particularly during increased intra-abdominal pressure.

MICTURITION CYCLE

FILLING PHASE

The urine produced by the kidneys is propelled along the ureters into the bladder by peristalsis activity of the smooth ureteric muscle. The viscoelastic bladder is compliant to the volume of urine produced so that the bladder pressure remains low. When the bladder fills to 350–500 ml, the intravesical stretch receptors are stimulated via S2–4 which trigger a strong desire to void. The first sensation of filling is usually at approximately 200 ml. This initial desire to void can normally be controlled and voiding will usually take place following a strong desire to void (Figure 4.1).

VOIDING PHASE

Voiding is initiated by the relaxation of the striated musculature under voluntary control and voiding is completed by reflex action. The detrusor muscle contracts increasing the internal pressure in the bladder. Urine passes through the relaxed involuntary and voluntary muscle of the urethra. Voiding occurs at approximately 15 ml/sec in the male (20 ml/sec in the female), although the rate is higher in young men. Maximum flow rates are obtained at volumes of 300 ml to 400 ml in normal men. Flow rate is improved by a standing position in men (Berger 1995). In healthy men, the bladder empties completely (Figure 4.2).

REFILLING PHASE

After micturition, the external urethral muscles and the pelvic floor muscles including the bulbocavernosus muscles contract whilst the detrusor

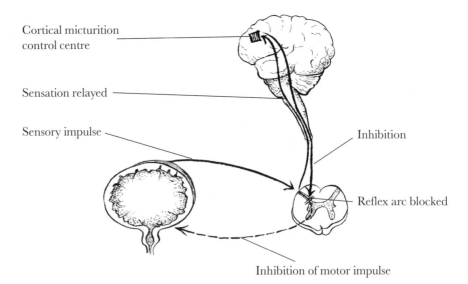

Figure 4.1. Bladder filling (Reproduced by permission of John Wiley & Sons. *Source*: Dorey, 2001b)

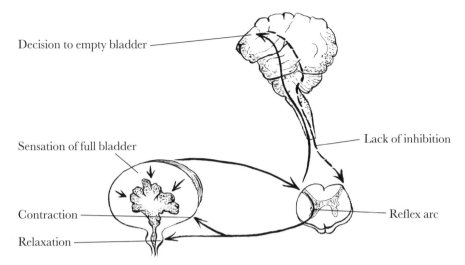

Figure 4.2. Bladder voiding (Reproduced by permission of John Wiley & Sons. *Source*: Dorey, 2001b)

muscle relaxes enabling the bladder to refill, thus repeating the micturition cycle.

NEUROLOGICAL CONTROL OF THE BLADDER

The neurological control of the bladder is a complex subject and the local interactions between neurologic modulators of the urethra and detrusor muscle are less clear (Gray 1996). The detrusor muscle and bladder neck sphincter are under neurological control from the peripheral nerves, spinal cord, pons, cerebral cortex and neurotransmitters of the lower urinary tract (Figure 4.3).

PERIPHERAL NERVES

The bladder is innervated by the pelvic nerves arising from the second, third and fourth sacral nerves (S2–4).

The levator ani, ischiococcygeus and bulbocavernosus are supplied by the perineal branch of the pudendal nerve (S2, 3, 4).

The nerve supply to the external urethral sphincter is from the pudendal nerve (S2, 3, 4).

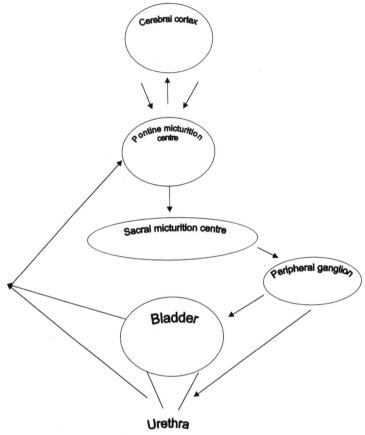

Figure 4.3. Neurological control of the bladder (Reproduced by permission of John Wiley & Sons. *Source*: Dorey, 2001b)

SPINAL CORD

Lower urinary tract function depends essentially on the integrity of the lumbo-sacral spinal cord. Controversy still exists concerning the role of the sacral micturition reflex centre. However, the sacral reflex is mediated by the pelvic and pudendal nerves and is subject to facilitation or inhibition by descending central nervous system pathways (Levin & Wein 1995).

SYMPATHETIC CONTROL

Bladder storage is partly under sympathetic control. Sympathetic stimulation of the bladder promotes detrusor relaxation and bladder filling via the afferent and efferent tracts arising between T10 and L2 spinal segments. The inferior hypogastric plexus provides sympathetic tone of the bladder neck and smooth muscle of the proximal urethra.

PARASYMPATHETIC CONTROL

Voiding is under parasympathetic control. Parasympathetic stimulation produces a detrusor contraction and urethral sphincter relaxation via the afferent and efferent tracts located in S2–4 pelvic plexus.

BRAIN

The frontal lobes of the cerebral cortex contain a detrusor motor area (Andrew & Nathan 1964). The thalamus may have an inhibitory effect on detrusor contractility (Gray 1998). The basal ganglia exert an inhibitory influence on the detrusor reflex allowing continence control. The hypothalamus may exert some influence but the function is unclear (Torrens 1987). The pontine micturition centre activates detrusor contraction and sphincteric co-ordination (Griffiths et al. 1990).

NEUROTRANSMITTERS

The detrusor muscle is a smooth muscle which contains actin and myosin filaments. It relies on calcium ions to contract (Steers 1992). The primary neurotransmitter acetylcholine is released under parasympathetic control causing a detrusor contraction and voiding, whereas noradrenaline under control of the sympathetic system is the primary neurotransmitter causing inhibition of the detrusor muscle and allowing storage to take place.

INTEGRAL BLADDER STORAGE AND VOIDING REFLEXES

Neurological integral reflexes control bladder storage and voiding. Spinal reflex control of the bladder and its sphincters are normally co-ordinated by brainstem mechanisms. Overactivity or functional failure of one or more integral reflexes may cause a significant disorder of the lower urinary tract function.

URINE STORAGE REFLEXES

During the storage of urine, distension of the bladder produces low-level vesical afferent firing, which in turn stimulates sympathetic outflow to the bladder base and urethra and pudendal outflow to the external urethral sphincter (Morrison et al. 2005). Sympathetic activity also inhibits bladder

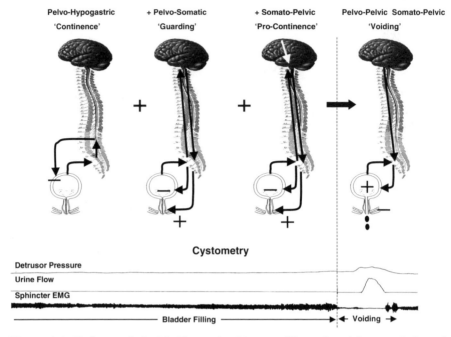

Figure 4.4. Reflexes of the bladder and sphincters (Reproduced by permission of Professor MD Craggs)

detrusor muscle contraction. These responses occur by spinal reflex pathways and are termed pelvo-hypogastric 'continence' and pelvo-somatic 'guarding' reflexes respectively. During exertion, when there is an increase in intra-abdominal pressure, the guarding reflex is further activated reflexly to prevent so-called 'stress' urinary incontinence. As the bladder approaches fullness the guarding reflex becomes strongly modulated by the pontine storage centre, the detrusor muscle becomes more inhibited, voluntary contractions of the sphincter and pelvic floor muscles are reinforced (the 'pro-continence response') and sensations of the desire to void are suppressed until a toilet can be found (Figure 4.4).

VOIDING REFLEXES

At an appropriate time, volitional effort switches the pontine storage centre 'off' causing the bladder neck and urethral sphincters to relax. Simultaneously, the pontine micturition centre is switched 'on' to activate the pelvo-pelvic 'voiding' reflex pathways. Intense bladder afferent firing now elicits a series of sacral reflexes which produce sustained parasympathetic outflow to contract the bladder detrusor muscle powerfully for efficient voiding.

SUMMARY

The continence mechanism in men consists of the bladder base, the bladder neck and the proximal urethra supplemented by the rhabdosphincter. Urinary continence relies on an intact urinary system with a competent urethral sphincter and integration of the neural modulatory structures in the peripheral nervous system, spinal cord, pons and cerebral cortex. Neurological urine-storage reflexes control storage of urine in the bladder and urine-voiding reflexes control micturition.

5 Prostate Conditions and their Treatment

Key points

- The most common prostate conditions are benign prostatic hyperplasia, prostate cancer and prostatitis.
- The prevalence of benign prostatic hyperplasia increases with age.
- Prostate cancer accounts for 1 in 10 deaths in Europe and North America.
- There are different classifications of prostatitis.

INVESTIGATIONS FOR PROSTATE CONDITIONS

Tests which assist in the diagnosis of benign prostatic hyperplasia and prostate cancer are:

1. Urinalysis of mid-stream urine to eliminate urinary infection.
2. Uroflow, to assess the flow rate during micturition. A reduced flow rate and a high residual volume of urine in the bladder may demonstrate blockage (Figure 5.1).
3. Estimation of volume of urine after voiding using ultrasound over the lower abdomen to test for retention of urine in the bladder.
4. Digital rectal examination, in side-lying or forward-bending to assess size and consistency of the prostate gland. Abnormal irregularities may be indicative of prostate cancer.
5. Prostate-specific antigen (PSA) blood test in men between 50 and 75 years of age. This test is not definitive but is used in conjunction with other tests.
6. Rectal ultrasound scan to aid the diagnosis of prostatic cancer and benign prostatic hyperplasia (BPH).
7. Urodynamics to diagnose sphincter/bladder dysfunction.
8. Flexible cystoscopy for the diagnosis of strictures, interstitial cystitis and bladder tumours.
9. X-ray of kidneys, ureters and bladder (KUB) for stones, bladder tumours and foreign bodies.
10. Intravenous pyelogram (IVP) to assess upper urinary tract problems.

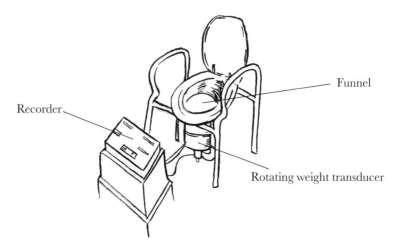

Recorder

Funnel

Rotating weight transducer

Figure 5.1. Uroflowmeter (Reproduced by permission of John Wiley & Sons. *Source*: Dorey, 2001b)

11. Cystogram to aid the diagnosis of bladder pathology.
12. Magnetic resonance to aid diagnosis of pelvic pathology.
13. Bladder diary to monitor amount and timing of fluid input and output.
14. Prostate biopsy via rectum to diagnose prostate cancer.

BENIGN PROSTATIC HYPERPLASIA

Benign prostatic hyperplasia (BPH) (Figure 5.2) is a condition which includes benign prostatic enlargement (BPE) due to a multiplication of normal cells, lower urinary tract symptoms (LUTS) and bladder outlet obstruction (BOO). The prevalence of BPE increases with age. In a study of 597 men by Simpson et al. (1996), the age-specific rates for BPE, using the threshold of a prostate size of over 20 g, was reported to be 62 % for men 40–49 years of age, 78 % for men 50–59 years of age, 89 % for men 60–69 years of age and 89 % for men 70–79 years of age. However, they found no significant relationship between prostate size and symptoms.

Pathologic BPH is divided into two stages: microscopic and macroscopic (Sant & Long 1994). The earliest microscopic nodules of BPH develop in men between 30 and 50 years of age in the periurethral zone and may infiltrate the transitional zone. The aetiology of BPH is imprecisely defined. Ageing and the presence of androgens, especially dihydrotestosterone, are essential factors for the development of BPH.

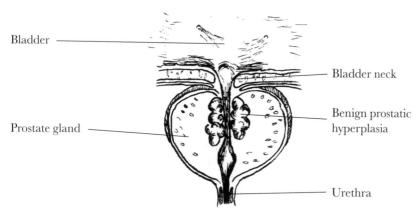

Bladder

Bladder neck

Benign prostatic
hyperplasia

Prostate gland

Urethra

Figure 5.2. Benign prostatic hyperplasia (Reproduced by permission of John Wiley & Sons. *Source*: Dorey, 2001b)

TREATMENT FOR BPH

Transurethral resection of prostate (TURP) is the most frequently performed operation for BPH and is performed using a resectoscope with a cutting loop and coagulating electrode. In all forms of prostatectomy, the bladder neck is resected rendering the closure mechanism incompetent. Postoperatively continence relies on the strength and integrity of the external urinary sphincter. Some men experience retrograde ejaculation after prostatectomy. During normal ejaculation, closure of the bladder neck prevents seminal fluid entering the bladder. However, post-surgery the seminal fluid enters the bladder and is voided at the next micturition.

A retropubic or suprapubic prostatectomy is occasionally performed for larger prostates with BPH. Surgery is performed through a lower abdominal incision. The prostate gland is surgically enucleated leaving the outer capsule intact.

The range of minimally invasive treatments for men with BPH has grown steadily in the last decade. The energy sources range from microwaves and radiofrequency waves to high-intensity focused ultrasound, laser vaporisation/coagulation/resection and electrosurgical techniques (Djavan et al. 1999). However, TURP is still considered the gold standard. A systematic review of six studies comparing laser to TURP was unable to make a definitive judgement about safety, efficacy and durability owing to the poor methodology of the studies (Wheelahan et al. 2000).

As an alternative to surgery, other treatments such as drug therapy and stents may be advised. Patients will be guided by their urologist to make an informed choice from the different treatments available.

There are two drug therapy treatments available for the reduction of urinary symptoms caused by benign prostatic enlargement (see Chapter 12).

For men with retention but who are unfit for surgery, wire or silicone mesh stents may be positioned inside the restricted prostatic urethra to allow the free flow of urine. Unfortunately, various problems can arise with the use of stents. They can cause infection and are prone to encrustation or even migration into the bladder.

PROSTATE CANCER

Prostate cancer is the commonest cancer in men in the UK, with over 24,700 new cases and 9,000 deaths a year (Cancer Research UK, 2005). In England and Wales, the incidence is 54.2 per 100,000 of population in males of all ages (Chamberlain et al. 1997) accounting for 1 in 10 deaths in Europe and North America (Kirby et al. 1994). In the UK, it accounts for 8,848 deaths a year (Office of Population Census and Surveys 1996). Prostate cancer occurs as the result of primary tumours in the majority of cases (Gray 1992). Prostate cancer is caused by a multiplication of abnormal cells. Cancer is associated with loss of apoptotic potential (where cells lose the ability to die) and uncontrolled proliferation (Denmeade et al. 1996). Prostate adenocarcinomas originate within the stroma (cortex) of the gland with a firm, single or multifocal nodule. As the tumour volume increases, it causes enlargement of the prostate gland, which may give rise to symptoms of bladder outlet obstruction. The cause of prostate adenocarcinoma remains unclear but genetic, racial, viral and dietary factors have been suggested (Figure 5.3).

Benign prostatic hyperplasia and prostate cancer are two separate entities. One does not lead to the other; however, they may co-exist. Prostate cancer may be slowly growing in the elderly patient, who may die 'with' rather than 'of' the disease.

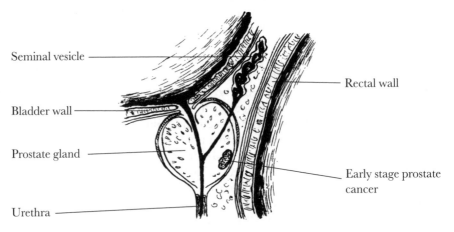

Figure 5.3. Prostate cancer (Reproduced by permission of John Wiley & Sons. *Source*: Dorey, 2001b)

TREATMENT OF PROSTATE CANCER

For prostate cancer, patients may be given the choice of a radical prostatectomy, radiotherapy (called brachytherapy if radioactive seeds are used), anti-androgen treatment or, more rarely now, orchidectomy. Shared decision-making is now considered to be an integral part of gaining informed consent from patients for most urological surgery. Emberton et al. (1997) have produced an interactive CD-ROM multi-media patient information package for men with lower urinary tract symptoms which can be used to aid decision-making. Radical prostatectomy is becoming increasingly preferred for localised disease, particularly now that nerve-sparing techniques can help to preserve potency and continence (Resnick 1992).

URETHRAL STRICTURE

Urethral stricture occurs when scar tissue narrows the urethra following urethritis or trauma. It may occur at any part of the urethra from the meatus (external opening) to the prostatic urethra. At the peno-scrotal junction, strictures form from traumatic catheterisation (Denning 1996).

Treatment for a stricture consists of dilatation under anaesthetic or surgical division by urethrotomy. Maintenance treatment may consist of regular dilatation by intermittent self-catheterisation (Lawrence & MacDonagh 1988).

SPHINCTEROTOMY

A sphincterotomy is an operation where the proximal sphincter at the bladder neck or the external urinary sphincter is cut to allow the passage of urine. Blockage is due to spasm of the sphincter, which occurs during detrusor/sphincter dyssynergia.

PROSTATITIS

There are different types of prostatitis which include acute bacterial, chronic bacterial and non-bacterial. Each type may cause considerable rectal and suprapubic discomfort (Chapter 7).

SUMMARY

There are a number of investigations which may assist in the diagnosis of benign prostate hyperplasia, prostate cancer and prostatitis. These three separate prostate conditions may co-exist. There are a number of treatment options for each condition.

6 Urinary Incontinence

Key points

- Urinary incontinence is defined as the complaint of any involuntary leakage of urine.
- The International Continence Society has classified urinary incontinence into different types.
- The prevalence of urinary incontinence ranges from 3.6 % in men 45 years old to 28.2 % in men 90 years old.

DEFINITION OF URINARY INCONTINENCE

Urinary incontinence is defined by the International Continence Society (ICS) as the complaint of any involuntary leakage of urine (Abrams et al. 2002). In each specific circumstance, urinary incontinence should be further described by specifying relevant factors such as type, frequency, severity, precipitating factors, social impact, effect on hygiene and quality of life, the measures used to contain the leakage, and whether or not the individual seeks or desires help because of urinary incontinence. The urinary incontinence conditions are defined by the presence of urodynamic observations associated with characteristic symptoms or signs and/or non-urodynamic evidence of relevant pathological processes (Abrams et al. 2002).

PREVALENCE OF URINARY INCONTINENCE IN MEN

The absolute incidence of urinary incontinence among men in the UK remains unknown. Urinary incontinence is an under-reported problem probably owing to social stigma (Gray 1992). Men may be too embarrassed to consult their doctors. Perhaps all patients should be questioned tactfully about their continence status when presenting to any medical professional. Many cases of urinary incontinence are transient, brought on by infection, immobility or acute disease. However, many others represent a chronic condition that persists until proper treatment and bladder management strategies allowing social continence are instituted (Gray 1992).

The prevalence of urinary incontinence in men increases with age and ranges from 3.6 % in men 45 years old to 28.2 % in men 90 years old or older

(Britton et al. 1990; Brocklehurst 1993; Malmsten et al. 1997; Thomas et al. 1980). The prevalence of reported urinary incontinence in men also varies with the definition of incontinence and the threshold of incontinence used. In many of the larger studies incontinence was defined in different ways, which made a true comparison impossible because of these inconsistencies. For example, Britton et al. (1990) found an incidence of 27 % in 578 men aged 60 to 85 years of age who attended a screening clinic in Leeds and completed a self-administered questionnaire. Incontinence was defined as 'Dribbling into pants at any time', whereas, Brocklehurst (1993) interviewed a random sample of 4,007 community dwelling adults, of whom 1,883 were men aged 30 and over, and used the definition of urinary incontinence as 'Any leaking, wet pants or damp pants?' and the threshold of 'Have you ever suffered from?'. The study revealed 6.6 % (124 men) had been incontinent of urine at some time. Of these, 60 % (74 men) were worried or concerned about their incontinence and almost 50 % experienced limitation of daily activities such as using public transport, visiting friends or going to work.

INCIDENCE OF URINARY INCONTINENCE FOLLOWING TRANSURETHRAL RESECTION OF THE PROSTATE

Transurethral resection of the prostate is one of the most frequently performed surgical procedures in the UK, with about 20 % of men over 50 years likely to undergo resection (Garraway et al. 1991). Every year about 50,000 men in Great Britain have prostate surgery (Office of Health Economics, 1995). A survey in England of 5,276 patients who had undergone TURP found that a third (1,759 men) who were continent before surgery reported some incontinence 3 months post-prostatectomy (Emberton et al. 1996). In a confidential questionnaire by the Royal College of Surgeons in England as part of the National Prostatectomy Audit, 6 % of patients who stated they were continent pre-TURP described severe incontinence or the use of pads 3 months after operation (Neal 1997).

INCIDENCE OF URINARY INCONTINENCE FOLLOWING RADICAL PROSTATECTOMY

Donnellan et al. (1997) reported 6 % mildly incontinent, 6 % moderately incontinent and 4 % severely incontinent at 1 year after radical prostatectomy. No patient reported pre-operative incontinence but, after surgery, urinary incontinence was reported to be the most distressing postoperative problem. Davidson et al. (1996) investigated 188 previously continent men following radical prostatectomy. They graded incontinence as Grade 1, those patients needing 1–2 pads per day, and Grade 2, those patients who needed 2 or more pads per day. They found that the amount of the initial loss did not predict the time to continence. The results for both grades combined showed that 107 (56 %) were incontinent postoperatively after catheter removal, 40 (21 %) were incontinent at 3 months and 24 (14 %) were still incontinent at 1 year. However, Rudy et al. (1984) reported incontinence following radical prostatectomy to be as high as 87 % at 6 months after surgery, based on strict urodynamic testing criteria. The definition of incontinence used was 'the occasional pad'. This paper was written prior to nerve-sparing surgery.

Koeman et al. (1996) used a self-administered questionnaire and reported that after radical prostatectomy 9 out of 14 men had involuntary loss of urine at orgasm, even though only one patient suffered from stress incontinence. Koeman et al. (1996) reported that the prevalence of this type of leakage may be higher than previously thought. Moul (1994) and Paulson (1991) both state that post-prostatectomy incontinence may be avoided by adhering to careful surgical technique.

CLASSIFICATION OF LOWER URINARY TRACT SYMPTOMS (Abrams et al. 2002a)

Symptoms are the subjective indicator of a disease or a change in condition as perceived by the patient, carer or partner and may lead him to seek help from a healthcare professional.

Lower urinary tract symptoms are divided into three groups: storage, voiding and post-micturition symptoms.

STORAGE SYMPTOMS

Storage symptoms are experienced during the storage phase of the bladder, and include daytime frequency and nocturia.

Increased daytime frequency is the complaint by the patient who considers that he voids too often by day.

Nocturia is the complaint that the individual has to wake at night one or more times to void.

Urgency is the complaint of a sudden compelling desire to pass urine, which is difficult to defer.

Stress urinary incontinence is the complaint of involuntary leakage on effort or exertion, or on sneezing or coughing. Stress urinary incontinence is almost always iatrogenic. Men at risk are those after radical prostatectomy, radiotherapy and, occasionally, transurethral resection of prostate (Figure 6.1).

Urge urinary incontinence is the complaint of the involuntary leakage accompanied by or immediately preceded by urgency. Urge urinary incontinence may be caused by detrusor overactivity which may be iatrogenic or neurogenic (Figure 6.2).

Mixed urinary incontinence is the complaint of involuntary leakage associated with urgency and also with exertion, effort, sneezing or coughing.

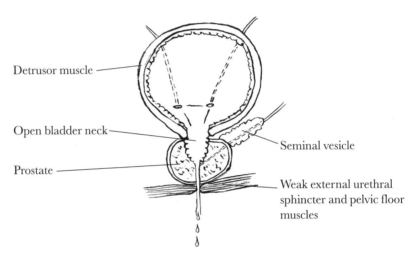

Figure 6.1. Stress urinary incontinence following transurethral resection of prostate (Reproduced by permission of John Wiley & Sons. *Source*: Dorey, 2001b)

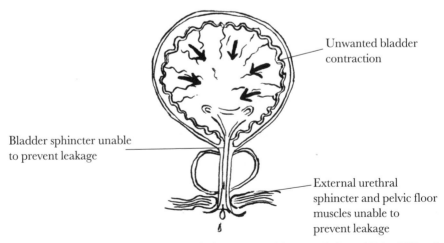

Figure 6.2. Urge urinary incontinence (Reproduced by permission of John Wiley & Sons. *Source*: Dorey, 2001b)

Nocturnal enuresis is the complaint of loss of urine occurring during sleep.

Continuous urinary incontinence is the complaint of continuous leakage.

VOIDING SYMPTOMS

Voiding symptoms are experienced during the voiding phase.

Slow stream is reported by the man as his perception of reduced urine flow, usually compared to previous performance or in comparison to others.

Intermittent stream (intermittency) is the term used when the man describes urine flow, which stops and starts, on one or more occasions, during micturition.

Hesitancy is the term used when a man describes difficulty in initiating micturition resulting in a delay in the onset of voiding after he is ready to pass urine.

Straining to void describes the muscular effort used to either initiate, maintain or improve the urinary stream.

Terminal dribble is the term used when a man describes a prolonged final part of micturition, when flow has slowed to a trickle/dribble.

POST-MICTURITION SYMPTOMS

Post-micturition symptoms are experienced immediately after micturition.

Feeling of incomplete emptying is a self-explanatory term for a feeling the man has after passing urine.

Post-micturition dribble should be distinguished from terminal dribble, which occurs at the end of micturition. It is a common problem for men of all ages (Pomfret 1993), but particularly troublesome in older men (Paterson et al. 1997). Post-micturition dribble is attributed to a failure of the bulbocavernosus muscle to evacuate the bulbar portion of the urethra (Feneley 1986; Millard 1989) causing pooling of urine in the bulbar urethra which can dribble with movement. Men who suffer from post-micturition dribble may prefer to wear pads or dribble collectors but an alternative treatment is pelvic floor muscle exercises (Paterson et al. 1997; Dorey et al. 2004b) (Chapter 9).

SIGNS SUGGESTIVE OF LOWER URINARY TRACT DYSFUNCTION (Abrams et al. 2002a)

Men can be asked to record micturitions and symptoms for a period of days to provide valuable information in three main forms:

1. *Micturition time chart* records only the times of micturitions, day and night, for at least 24 hours.
2. *Frequency/volume chart* records the volumes voided as well as the time of each micturition, day and night, for at least 24 hours.
3. *Bladder diary* records the times of micturitions and voided volumes, incontinence episodes, pad usage and other information such as fluid intake, the degree of urgency and the degree of incontinence.

The following measurements can be abstracted from frequency/volume charts and bladder diaries.

Daytime frequency is the number of voids recorded during waking hours and includes the last void before sleep and the first void after waking and rising in the morning.

Nocturia is the number of voids recorded during a night's sleep: each void is preceded and followed by sleep. Nocturia can be regarded as a symptom, a condition and/or a feature of nocturnal polyuria (Van Kerrebroeck & Weiss 1999). Nocturia can be assessed using the nocturia index and dividing the nightly voided urine volume by the functional bladder capacity (Table 6.1). The key factors associated with nocturia are summarised in Table 6.2.

24-hour frequency is the total number of daytime voids and episodes of nocturia during a specified 24-hour period.

24-hour production is measured by collecting all urine for 24 hours.

Polyuria is defined as the measured production of more than 2.8 litres of urine in 24 hours in adults. The figure of 2.8 litres is based on a 70-kg man voiding >40 ml/kg.

Table 6.1. Definitions of the classification and aetiology of nocturia (Reproduced by permission of Blackwell Publishing Ltd. *Source*: Kerrebroeck & Weiss, 1999)

Variable	Definition
Nocturnal urine volume (NUV)	Nightly voided volume plus first morning voided volume
Functional bladder capacity (FBC)	Largest single recorded voided volume from 24-hour voiding diary
Nocturia Index (NI)	$\dfrac{NUV}{FBC}$
Actual number of nightly voids (ANV)	Recorded from bladder diary
Predicted number of nightly voids (PNV)	NI minus 1 (rounded to next highest integer if this is not a whole number)
Nocturnal bladder capacity index (NBCI)	ANV minus PNV; if PNV > ANV then NBCI = 0
Nocturnal polyuria index (NPI)	$\dfrac{NUV}{\text{24-hour total voided volume}}$ (normal <35%)

Nocturnal urine volume is defined as the total volume of urine passed between the time the man goes to bed with the intention of sleeping and the time of waking with the intention of rising. It excludes the last void before going to bed but includes the first void after rising in the morning.

Nocturnal polyuria is present when an increased proportion of the 24-hour output occurs at night (normally during the 8 hours while the man is in bed). It excludes the last void before sleep but includes the first void in the morning. Nocturnal polyuria is present when greater than 20 % (in young adults) to 33 % (in men over 65 years) is produced at night. Nocturia increases with advancing age. By the eighth decade 80 % of men get up at least once a night or more to void (Middlekoop et al. 1996). However there are many reasons for nocturnal polyuria (see Table 5.3). Nocturnal polyuria can be assessed using the nocturnal polyuria index (NPI) and dividing the nocturnal urine volume (NUV) by the 24-hour total voided urine volume (Table 6.1).

Maximum voided volume is the largest volume of urine voided during a single micturition and is determined either from the frequency/volume chart or bladder diary.

Table 6.2. Major factors associated with nocturia (Reproduced with permission of Blackwell Publishing Ltd. *Source*: Fonda, 1999)

Ageing
Psychogenic
Behavioural
Sleep changes, disturbance and amount of time spent in bed
Polyuria syndromes
Bladder problems
Neurological causes
Combinations of all of the above

Table 6.3. Causes of nocturnal polyuria (Reproduced with permission of Blackwell Publishing Ltd. *Source*: Van Kerrebroeck & Weiss, 1999)

Cause	Reason
Reverse nocturnal/diurnal urine production	Absence of circadian rhythmicity in arginine vasopressin (AVP) secretion: solute diuresis mediated by increased atrial natriuretic peptide (ANP) levels in patients with sleep apnoea
Polydipsia (excessive thirst)	Polyuria
	Diabetes mellitus/insipidus
	Excessive fluid intake, especially in the evening
Third-space fluid loss	Congestive heart failure
	Venous insufficiency
	Excessive salt intake
	Hypoalbuminaemia/nephrotic syndrome
Other	Late evening administration of drinks

Urinary incontinence (the sign) is defined as urine leakage seen during examination: this may be urethral or extra-urethral.

Stress urinary incontinence is the observation of voluntary leakage from the urethra, synchronous with exertion/effort, or sneezing or coughing.

Extra-urethral incontinence is defined as the observation of urine leakage through channels other than the urethra.

Uncategorised incontinence is the observation of involuntary leakage that cannot be classified into one of the categories on the basis of signs and symptoms.

URODYNAMIC TERMINOLOGY (Abrams et al. 2002a)

Normal detrusor function allows bladder filling with little or no change in pressure. No involuntary phasic contractions occur despite provocation.

Detrusor overactivity is a urodynamic observation characterised by involuntary detrusor contractions during the filling phase which may be spontaneous or provoked.

Phasic detrusor overactivity is defined by a characteristic wave form and may or may not lead to urinary incontinence.

Terminal detrusor overactivity is defined as a single involuntary detrusor contraction occurring at cystometric capacity, which cannot be suppressed, and results in incontinence usually resulting in bladder emptying (voiding).

Detrusor overactivity incontinence is incontinence due to an involuntary detrusor contraction.

Detrusor overactivity may also be qualified, when possible, to cause: *neurogenic detrusor overactivity* when there is a relevant neurological condition; *idiopathic detrusor overactivity* when there is no defined cause.

Detrusor underactivity is defined as a contraction of reduced strength and/or duration, resulting in prolonged bladder emptying and/or a failure to achieve complete bladder emptying within a normal time span.

Acontractile detrusor is one that cannot be demonstrated to contract during urodynamic studies.

Post-void residual is defined as the volume of urine left in the bladder at the end of micturition.

Urodynamic stress incontinence is noted during filling cystometry, and is defined as the involuntary leakage of urine during increased abdominal pressure, in the absence of a detrusor contraction.

Detrusor sphincter dyssynergia is defined as a detrusor contraction concurrent with an involuntary contraction of the urethral and/or periurethral striated muscle. Occasionally flow may be prevented altogether. It may occur in men with a high spinal cord injury. The smooth muscle of the bladder neck may also be responsible.

NOCTURNAL ENURESIS

The symptom nocturnal enuresis is the complaint of urinary loss which occurs only during sleep (Blaivas et al. 1997). The cause remains obscure. Hereditary factors, sleep disturbance and natriuresis (excretion of sodium ions) may play a part but remain unproven. In children enuresis may be caused by incomplete bladder emptying. There are similarities between enuresis and nocturia where both entities are based on nocturnal polyuria with urine production exceeding the bladder capacity. The absence of a circadian rhythm in arginine vasopressin (AVP) is also associated with both enuresis and nocturia (Djurhuus et al. 1999).

INCONTINENCE ASSOCIATED WITH RETENTION

Incontinence of urine may be associated with over-distension of the bladder caused by obstruction, detrusor underactivity or impaired contractility.

UNCONSCIOUS INCONTINENCE

Unconscious incontinence may occur in the absence of urge and without conscious recognition of the urinary loss.

FUNCTIONAL INCONTINENCE

The ICS classification fails to recognise functional incontinence as a type of incontinence. Functional incontinence occurs when men are unable to get to the bathroom in time due to mobility and dexterity problems. Functional problems frequently mask the real cause of the incontinence or, conversely, functional incontinence may be caused by an inability to reach the toilet in time. This can be a most distressing problem for the elderly and immobile who would be continent without their handicap.

SUMMARY

The International Continence Society has standardised the terminology in the classification of urinary incontinence. The most common types of incontinence in men are stress urinary incontinence, urge urinary incontinence and post-micturition dribble.

7 Pelvic Pain in Men

Key points

- Acute pelvic pain in men may be caused by infection, physical or iatrogenic trauma, or neurological involvement.
- Chronic pelvic pain syndromes include painful bladder and urethral, scrotal, perineal and pelvic pain syndromes.
- A multidisciplinary approach using analgesics, physiotherapy and psychological interventions may be indicated.
- Various physiotherapeutic approaches include relaxation, trunk stability, posture, manual techniques, general exercise and electrotherapy.

INTRODUCTION

Pelvic pain, discomfort and pressure are part of the abnormal sensations felt by an individual with lower urinary tract symptoms (Abrams et al. 2002). Pain may or may not be related to bladder filling or voiding. Pain should be characterised by type, location, frequency, duration, and precipitating and relieving factors. Pelvic pain may be acute or chronic.

DEFINITIONS OF PELVIC PAIN

The ICS terminology for genital and lower urinary tract pain recognises different types of pain (Abrams et al. 2002):

- *Bladder pain* is felt suprapubically or retropubically, usually increasing with bladder filling, and may persist after voiding.
- *Urethral pain* is felt in the urethra and the man indicates the urethra as the site.
- *Scrotal pain* may or may not be localised, for example to the testis, epididymis, cord structures or scrotal skin.
- *Perineal pain* in men is felt between the scrotum and the anus. Perineal pain may be present in patients with orchialgia (pain in one or both testicles) and non-bacterial prostatitis (Wesselmann et al. 1997).

- *Pelvic pain* is less well defined than, for example, bladder, urethral or peri-neal pain and is less clearly related to the micturition cycle or to bowel function and is not localised to any single pelvic organ.

ACUTE PELVIC PAIN

Acute pain may affect any of the pelvic structures from nerve involvement in response to underlying pathology from infection, physical trauma or surgery. It may be relieved if the underlying cause is treated (Gee et al. 1990).

CHRONIC PELVIC PAIN SYNDROMES

Chronic pelvic pain is a complex problem in men and may involve the pelvic floor muscles (Knight 2005). Chronic pelvic pain syndrome endures for 6 months or more and therefore differs from acute pain. Chronic pelvic pain is a sensory, behavioural and psychological process that results from persistent nociceptor input and involves different pathways from those activated in acute pain situations (Steege 1998).

Genito-urinary pain syndromes are imprecise diagnoses of varying combi-nations of symptoms with chronic pain as the major complaint but concomi-tant complaints are of lower urinary tract, bowel and sexual nature (Abrams et al. 2002). These syndromes include painful bladder syndrome, urethral pain syndrome, scrotal pain syndrome, perineal pain syndrome and pelvic pain syndrome. In each case there is no proven infection or other obvious pathology. Genito-urinary pain syndromes are well described but under-recognised and poorly understood (Wesselmann et al. 1997).

Pain can accompany acute retention of urine which is defined as a painful, palpable or percussible bladder when the patient is unable to pass urine (Abrams et al. 2002).

Interstitial cystitis causes bladder pain and is a specific diagnosis and requires confirmation by typical cystoscopic and histological features (Abrams et al. 2002).

PENILE PAIN

Penile pain may be caused by penile prosthesis surgery, intracavernosal injec-tions and circumcision and may have a psychological aspect (Wesselmann et al. 1997). There have not been any psychological studies of penile pain which are independent of other urogenital pain disorders. Conditions causing penile pain are paraphimosis (constriction of the glans penis by a tight fore-skin), Peyronie's disease (penile deformity caused by fibrous tissue plaques which develop in the cavernous tissues), priapism (prolonged, painful penile erection lasting more than 4 hours) and herpes genitalis.

PROSTATITIS

Pelvic pain may be caused by prostatitis. Prostatitis is classified by the National Institutes of Health (Kreiger et al. 1999) as:

- Category I   Acute bacterial prostatitis
- Category II   Chronic bacterial prostatitis
- Category III   Chronic prostatitis/Chronic pelvic pain syndrome
- Category IIIA Inflammatory
- Category IIIB Non-bacterial prostatitis (formerly called prostatodynia)
- Category IV   Asymptomatic inflammatory prostatitis

Prostatitis occurs as a result of inflammation of the glandular portion of the prostate (Gray 1992) causing discomfort in the rectal and suprapubic areas. The semen may be yellow or blood-stained. The symptoms of prostatitis may be malaise and fever in the acute stage before the onset of dysuria, urgency, frequency and obstructive voiding. In both the acute and chronic stages, there may be pelvic pain.

SEXUAL PAIN

Sexual pain is any pain that affects the ability to gain and maintain an erection and achieve orgasm and ejaculation. It may be due to urethritis, prostatitis, blockage to the seminal vesicles, and/or hypertonic pelvic floor muscles. An anal fissure can cause anal pain and is linked to erectile dysfunction (Shafik & El-Sibai 2000).

PAINFUL EJACULATION

Painful ejaculation is defined as pain during ejaculation (Ralph & Wylie 2005). In an internet survey of 163 men with prostatitis, 69 % reported pain before or after ejaculation (Roehrborn et al. 2003). This uncommon problem may have psychological or organic causes. Organic causes may be prostatitis or, less commonly, ejaculatory duct obstruction, inflammation or stones (Ralph & Wylie 2005).

INCIDENCE OF PELVIC PAIN

A mail questionnaire sent to 2,987 men aged 20 to 74 years was completed by 868 (29 %) men aged 52.1 ± 13.5 years (Nickel et al. 2001). Overall 187 (21.5 %) men reported an index pain score of 4 or greater on a scale of 0–10. Among these, there were 57 (6.6 %) men who had perineal and/or ejaculatory pain or discomfort and an index pain score of 8 or greater.

AETIOLOGY OF ACUTE PELVIC PAIN

Acute pelvic pain in men may be caused by infection or physical trauma, or may have iatrogenic or neurological causes.

INFECTION

Acute bacterial prostatitis occurs as a result of bacteria ascending via the urethra and is a cause of pelvic pain. An anal abscess may give rise to acute anal pain.

PHYSICAL TRAUMA

Falling backwards on the coccyx can cause an acute pain on sitting called coccygodynia. Fissures or severe haemorrhoids may cause spasm of the external anal sphincter and the severe anal pain may compromise the normal erection process.

Anodyspareunia can be defined as painful receptive anal intercourse (Rosser et al. 1998). Psychophysiological factors predicting anal pain during receptive anal intercourse are inadequate lubrication, inability to relax, and lack of digitoproctic stimulation. Greater pain can be caused by increased depth, rate of thrusting and lack of social comfort (Rosser et al. 1998).

Unwanted anal penetration from sexual abuse can cause anal pain and permanent internal anal sphincter and in some men external anal sphincter damage (Engel et al. 1995).

IATROGENIC CAUSES

Urological and rectal surgery may cause adhesions and scar tissue, which may entrap the pudendal nerve.

In a study of 239 patients, mean age 62 years (SD 13), who completed a questionnaire 39 months (SD 20.8) after retropubic radical prostatectomy, pain occurred during orgasm in 14 % of men (Barnas et al. 2004). This pain occurred in the penis (63 %), abdomen (9 %), rectum (24 %), and other areas (4 %). It occurred always (33 %), frequently (13 %), occasionally (35 %) and rarely (19 %).

NEUROLOGICAL CAUSES

Spinal cord and nerve root compression from spinal tumours, disc protrusion, tethered dura mater, or apophyseal joint dysfunction can refer pain to the pelvic region.

AETIOLOGY OF CHRONIC PELVIC PAIN

Chronic pelvic pain in men may be caused by chronic prostatitis, musculo-skeletal conditions, pelvic floor hypertonus, neurological conditions, visceral conditions and psychological factors.

CHRONIC PROSTATITIS

Chronic prostatitis may have a bacterial cause as a result of bacteria ascending via the urethra or it may be caused by a non-bacterial inflammation of the prostate and urethra. The causal agents of non-bacterial prostatitis have not been identified. Misdiagnosis is common as painful intrapelvic muscles can produce symptoms similar to those of prostatitis (Simons et al. 1999). In a sample of 103 men with voiding dysfunction and pelvic pain, researchers found that 83 % of men had tenderness and hypertonus in the pelvic floor muscles (Zermann et al. 2001).

MUSCULOSKELETAL CONDITIONS

Malfunction of the musculoskeletal pelvic girdle and spinal–pelvic dysfunctions can cause pelvic pain from poor posture and muscle imbalance. Poor posture may lead to visceral displacement, fibrosis of the fascia, shortened muscles and ligaments, and muscle spasm which may compromise pelvic nerves and blood vessels.

PELVIC FLOOR MUSCLE HYPERTONUS

Pelvic pain can be caused by pelvic floor muscle spasm. Muscle spasm causing chronic pain may be found in any of the pelvic floor muscles. It may be poorly localised. Trigger points in intrapelvic muscles can produce symptoms similar to those of prostatitis (pain between the anus and testicles) and misdiagnosis is common (Simons et al. 1999). Spasm of the puborectalis muscle causes puborectalis syndrome with difficulties in voiding faeces leading to constipation (Wasserman 1964). Spasm of the anal sphincter causes the sharp anal pain of proctalgia fugax (Schuster 1990). Perineal pain may be present in patients with orchialgia and non-bacterial prostatitis (Wesselmann et al. 1997).

NEUROLOGICAL CONDITIONS

Spinal conditions such as lumbar disc prolapse and apophyseal joint dysfunction can refer pain to the pelvic area. Compression and tethering of the dura mater from poor posture and tension causes compression of the spinal cord, nerve root stretching and blood vessel compression. This in turn may compromise normal bladder function and refer pain to the pelvic region.

The pudendal nerve runs through Alcock's canal and is vulnerable to traction and compression along its course giving rise to the perineal pain of pudendal neuralgia (Bensignor et al. 1996). This neuralgia is characterised by burning along the nerve distribution. Robert et al. (1993) stated that surgical transposition of the pudendal nerve may reduce pain.

VISCERAL CONDITIONS

Pelvic pain may be due to irritable bowel syndrome and interstitial cystitis which may co-exist with pelvic floor muscle hypertonus.

PSYCHOLOGICAL FACTORS

Psychological issues related to lifestyle including stress can cause physiological pelvic floor muscle spasm which may become a chronic condition due to a cycle of tension and pain.

ASSESSMENT OF PELVIC PAIN

A holistic approach should be used to identify the many possible factors contributing to pelvic pain. Subjective assessment should include marking a body diagram with painful areas using a 0–10 pain scale. Objective assessment should screen the spine, hips and pelvic joints for sources of pain. Superficial examination can identify hypertonus and painful trigger points in the superficial transverse perineal muscles and the external anal sphincter. Anal examination can identify hypertonus and trigger points in the puborectalis and pubococcygeus muscles.

TREATMENT OF ACUTE PELVIC PAIN

Bacterial prostatitis is treated with antibiotics.

Acute pain post-surgery is treated with analgesics. Occasionally haematomas need draining and scar tissue strictures need stretching or dividing.

Penile pain caused by penile prosthesis surgery, intracavernosal injections and circumcision may be relieved if the underlying cause is treated (Gee et al. 1990). The psychological aspect may also need psychological input.

TREATMENT OF CHRONIC PELVIC PAIN

Chronic bacterial prostatitis is treated with antibiotics.

A multidisciplinary approach using analgesics, physiotherapy and psychological interventions such as psychology and sex therapy may be indicated for chronic pelvic pain relief in men (Wesselmann et al. 1997). Various physiotherapeutic approaches include relaxation, trunk stability, posture, manual techniques, general exercise and electrotherapy.

BIOFEEDBACK

The main goal of physiotherapy is to rehabilitate the pelvic floor by increasing awareness and proprioception of the muscles so that the patient can discriminate between muscle spasm and muscle relaxation. The physiological response to stress is increased muscular tone or muscle hypertension. This increased tension can be associated with pelvic pain. Biofeedback can help to show the resting tone of the pelvic floor muscles on a screen. Biofeedback is the technique by which information about a normally unconscious physiological process is presented to the patient and/or the therapist as a visual, auditory or tactile signal (Abrams et al. 2002). Concentric pelvic floor contraction exercises should be discouraged until pelvic floor muscles have been lengthened by manual techniques and have the ability to relax (FitzGerald & Kotarinos 2003).

Chronic lower urinary tract symptoms in young men are often misdiagnosed as non-bacterial prostatitis. Kaplan et al. (1997) performed urodynamic studies on 43 men, 23 to 50 years old, with misdiagnosed chronic prostatitis and found contraction of the external urinary sphincter during voiding (pseudodyssynergia) to be the cause of functional bladder outlet obstruction. Six months of behaviour modification and biofeedback was successful in decreasing symptoms in 35 of these patients (83 %). Without a control group it is impossible to say how many men would have naturally improved during that time.

RELAXATION

Proctalgia fugax produces acute painful spasm of the external anal sphincter which can be alleviated by sitting on the toilet and bearing down gently as if to void faeces. This causes relaxation of the anal sphincter and may also release a small pellet of faecal matter trapped in the anal canal.

Relaxation and stress management may help those men who have stressful jobs, lifestyles and relationship difficulties. It may help men to visit a counsellor or a psychologist.

TRUNK STABILITY

Trunk stability is necessary for the interaction between the pelvic floor muscles and transversus abdominis. Trunk stability is also necessary for lumbar and pelvic joint realignment and serves to work the hip and trunk muscles especially multifidus. Muscle balance around the hip joint may be encouraged for inactive men, many of whom may have limited hip rotation.

POSTURE

Posture correction in sitting and standing and during daily activities may help to avoid the strain placed on the spine from poor posture. Habitual poor posture leads to muscle and ligament shortening and in the opposite muscles, lengthening and weakening. There is less strain on the spinal joints if they are held in a neutral position.

MANUAL TECHNIQUES

Manual techniques may be used to treat men with pelvic pain. Soft tissue mobilisation, myofascial release, visceral mobilisation, CranioSacral Therapy, Proprioceptive Neuromuscular Facilitation and lymphatic drainage may all have a role to play depending on the cause of the pain (Shelly et al. 2002). Soft tissue mobilisation is gentle massage and gentle stretching used to mobilise the skin, fascia and muscles which may be bound down, shortened and immobile due to pain, spasm and scarring. Thiele first reported massage to the pubococcygeus muscles through the rectum for coccygodynia (Thiele 1937). Myofascial release is a gentle manual technique aimed at muscles, ligaments and their fascial coverings to identify and treat trigger points responsible for referred pain. Anderson et al. (1999) found in 23 men with chronic non-bacterial prostatitis syndrome that weekly myofascial release significantly improved pain scores. Proprioceptive Neuromuscular Facilitation enables patients to feel when a muscle is stretched and recognise when it is contracting and when it is relaxed (Knott & Voss 1968). It is a physiotherapy treatment where manual resistance, in addition to different afferent stimuli, is used to facilitate motor function and decrease hypertonus (Claesson et al. 1999). CranioSacral Therapy is a gentle 'hands on' approach used to facilitate the body's ability to realign the spine, remove areas of tethering and compression to the dura mater, spinal cord, nerve roots and their sleeves. Because it acts on the deepest structures and organs of the nervous system, CranioSacral Therapy influences motor, pain and co-ordination mechanisms, the digestive system, heart function and the endocrine system (Upledger 2005). Lymphatic drainage is massage which is used to drain the venous and lymphatic vessels in the area and improve a sluggish blood supply.

GENERAL EXERCISE

General aerobic exercise helps cardiovascular function, increases circulation and decreases stress and depression and helps to relieve pain due to the release of endorphins. Those men who do not take regular exercise can be encouraged to spend part of each day walking and gradually increase exercise tolerance levels by walking up hills. Swimming and various sporting activities such as golf can help to increase adrenaline and give men the feel-good factor.

ELECTROTHERAPY

Hayden (1993) and Holland et al. (1994) treated orchialgia with transcutaneous electrical nerve stimulation (TENS) and considered the treatment beneficial.

PSYCHOLOGICAL INTERVENTIONS

Men who have pain and relationship difficulties, guilt, depression, anxieties, previous unpleasant experiences and sexual abuse may benefit by a referral to a psychologist or sex therapist.

PAIN FROM CANCER

It is important to note that there are no symptoms with prostate and bladder cancer in the early stages. The first sign of bladder cancer is haematuria. No two cancers are the same. In the later stages of prostate cancer there are symptoms of hip, leg and back pain, which may be mistaken for arthritis.

SUMMARY

Acute pelvic pain in men may be caused by infection or physical trauma, or may arise from iatrogenic or neurological causes. Chronic pelvic pain in men may be linked to chronic prostatitis, musculoskeletal conditions, pelvic floor muscle hypertonus, neurological conditions, visceral conditions and psychogenic factors.

A multidisciplinary approach using analgesics, physiotherapy and psychological interventions may be indicated for chronic pelvic pain relief in men. Various physiotherapeutic approaches include relaxation, trunk stability, posture, manual techniques, general exercise and electrotherapy.

8 Patient Assessment

Key points

- A detailed subjective and objective assessment is necessary in order to make a diagnosis.
- Urinalysis, uroflow and post-void residual tests contribute to the diagnosis.
- A digital anal assessment will reveal the strength and endurance of the pelvic floor muscles.

INTRODUCTION

Before a diagnosis can be made, and before treatment can be commenced, a subjective and objective assessment is required.

SUBJECTIVE ASSESSMENT

The subjective assessment is based on the patient's account of his symptoms. The Male Continence Assessment Form is in the Appendix. The subjective assessment should include questions in the following categories.

PATIENT DETAILS

Patient details should include the patient's age, occupation, hobbies and physical activities in order to make a lifestyle evaluation. Potential risk factors are immobility from a sedentary lifestyle or the strain from heavy or repeated lifting.

SURGICAL HISTORY

It is necessary to know the dates and outcomes of transurethral resection of prostate (TURP) and any repeat TURPs, radical prostatectomy, radiotherapy, urethral stricture division and any other abdominal or bowel surgery.

MAIN PROBLEM

It is necessary to have knowledge of the severity and duration of the main problem, the limitation of activities, quality of life (QoL) and bothersome rating (0–10) caused by the main problem.

SYMPTOMS

The following questions should be asked to ascertain the presenting symptoms. Does the man have leakage on exertion with symptoms of stress incontinence? What are the provoking factors, such as coughing, sneezing, shouting, rising from sitting and bending? Are there any bladder storage symptoms of urgency, urge incontinence, frequency and nocturia? How many times a night does the patient get up to void urine? Does he have nocturnal enuresis and wet the bed? In order to have knowledge of voiding (obstructive) symptoms, questions should be asked concerning the flow of urine. Does he have difficulty starting and maintaining the stream, and is the stream weaker than normal, or intermittent? Are the voided volumes small? At the end of the stream is there a terminal dribble? Does the bladder feel empty after micturition? Does he have to perform a Credé manoeuvre by leaning forwards and pressing on the lower abdomen whilst straining to void urine? Does he have to double void? Can he feel when he is voiding and is he aware when he is leaking? When he walks away from the toilet, is there an after-dribble called post-micturition dribble? Does he have a constant dribble of urine? Is it painful to pass urine? Any indication of pain in the pelvic area may be marked on a body chart. Is the urine dark, smelly, smoky or does it contain blood?

DURATION AND SEVERITY OF SYMPTOMS

The duration of each symptom needs to be noted plus the improvement or deterioration to date. The severity of each symptom can be marked on a visual analogue scale (0–10) indicating from 0 = no problem to 10 = severe problem.

AMOUNT OF LEAKAGE

The amount of leakage may be ascertained from a description by the patient and may be described as a few drops, or a medium or large leakage, the number of pads used per day, their size and whether the pads are damp, wet or soaked. Does the patient have an appliance and leg bag, use intermittent catheterisation or have an indwelling catheter?

FREQUENCY OF LEAKAGE

What is the frequency of leakage: is it daily, once a week or once a month? When does the leakage occur? Is the leakage provoked by: coughing, sneezing, shouting, walking, moving, running water, caffeine, alcohol, medications or some other trigger?

URINE STOP TEST

Can the patient stop or slow down the flow of urine mid-stream? This question provides the opportunity to explain that this exercise can lead to retention of urine and therefore should not be practised. Stopping mid-stream mimics detrusor dyssynergia, when the bladder and the sphincter are contracting at the same time.

BOWEL ACTIVITY

Does the patient suffer from constipation, strain to defaecate or practise digital evacuation? How many times a week does defaecation occur? Are the faeces liquid, soft or firm? Is there faecal urgency, faecal incontinence or incontinence of flatus? Does the patient use laxatives and does he have a balanced diet with sufficient fluids?

MEDICAL HISTORY

Has the patient suffered from prostatitis: how often and was it acute or chronic? Has he had acute or chronic cystitis and what is it like now? Is he allergic to latex and does he run the risk of anaphylactic shock if the therapist uses latex gloves? There is a significant correlation between latex sensitisation, and the number and duration of surgical procedures and intermittent catheterisations (De Castro et al. 1999). Does he have any metal implants such as a total hip replacement? Electrical stimulation is contraindicated if there is metal in the field, which may concentrate the current and produce a burn. Does he smoke, have respiratory problems and a cough exacerbating his incontinence? Does he take anticholinergic medication (tolterodine or oxybutinin), alpha-blockers such as doxazosin mesylate (Cardura), 5-alpha inhibitors, anti-androgen treatment or any other medication? What is the effect, and side-effects, of the medication? Has he undergone or is he undergoing radiotherapy? Is there a neurological problem such as diabetes, multiple sclerosis or Parkinson's disease, or a severe cervical or lumbar spine problem with a neurological deficit?

Previous treatment

Has the patient had previous conservative treatment and what was the outcome?

Body mass index

What is the patient's height and weight and what is his body mass index (BMI)? BMI = Weight in kilograms divided by height in metres squared. BMI > 25 = overweight; BMI > 30 = seriously overweight; BMI > 41 = dangerously overweight.

Sexual problems

Does the patient have difficulty gaining or maintaining penile erection? Does he wake with an erection? Does he have premature ejaculation?

Functional factors

Is the patient able to stand for urination? Does he have adequate mobility and dexterity? Are there any environmental problems which make access to the toilet difficult? Is he cognitively impaired or having psychological problems? Is there a patient support network of carers?

Motivation

Does the patient have the ability and motivation to incorporate the therapy into his lifestyle in order to comply with an exercise programme or with lifestyle changes.

MEDICAL INVESTIGATIONS

A full assessment includes a urinalysis of mid-stream urine to eliminate urinary infection; a uroflow, to monitor the strength of the stream during micturition; and a bladder ultrasound post-void residual examination to exclude urine retention. Other tests of interest are: prostate-specific antigen (PSA); urodynamics to diagnose genuine stress incontinence, detrusor overactivity and a low compliance bladder; and flexible cystoscopy for the diagnosis of strictures and bladder tumours. A 24-hour pad test is useful prior to treatment and then at discharge as an outcome measure.

BLADDER DIARY

A bladder diary records more than the conventional frequency/volume chart. The bladder diary records the times of micturitions and voided volumes, incontinence episodes, pad usage and other information such as fluid intake, the degree of urgency and the degree of incontinence (Abrams et al. 2002b). This diary provides information concerning: frequency of voiding, maximum voided volume, minimum voided volume, daily amount of fluid intake, amount of caffeine and alcohol intake, daily amount of urinary output, time of going to bed, amount voided at night, frequency of leakage, and number of pads used per day. The time that diuretic therapy is taken should be marked on the diary. The bladder diary confirms the diagnosis of urge incontinence, usually with attendant frequency and nocturia, and/or stress incontinence (Tables 8.1 and 8.2).

The bladder diary should be completed for at least 24 hours. It can be repeated at intervals to show progress.

Table 8.1. Bladder diary of a man with stress urinary incontinence (Reproduced by permission of John Wiley & Sons. *Source*: Dorey, 2001b)

Name _____ **Date** _____

Time	Tick voiding urine	Amount voided in ml	Tick leak	Type of drink	Amount drunk in ml	Pad change	Comments 'almost dry' 'damp' 'wet' or 'soaked'
6 am	✓	470	✓	Tea	250		Walked to bathroom – wet
7 am							
8 am	✓						
9 am							
10 am	✓	260		Coffee	250		
11 am							
12 am							
1 pm	✓	250		Soup	150		
2 pm							
3 pm			✓			✓	Lifted rubbish – wet
4 pm	✓	200		Tea	200		
5 pm							
6 pm	✓	200					
7 pm				Wine	250		
8 pm				Coffee	200		
9 pm							
10 pm			✓	Water	200	✓	Coughed – damp
11 pm	✓	350					
12 pm							
1 am							
2 am							
3 am							
4 am							
5 am							
Totals	7	1,730	3		1,500	2	

Please bring your completed diary with you to your next appointment

Table 8.2. Bladder diary of a man with urge urinary incontinence (Reproduced by permission of John Wiley & Sons. *Source*: Dorey, 2001b)

Name _____   **Date** _____

Time	Tick voiding urine	Amount voided in ml	Tick leak	Type of drink	Amount drunk in ml	Pad change	Comments 'almost dry' 'damp' 'wet' or 'soaked'
6 am	✓	130	✓	Tea	250		Rushed to bathroom
7 am	✓	150					
8 am	✓	50		Tea	250		
9 am	✓	80					
10 am	✓✓	100	✓	Coffee	250	✓	Urgency – wet
11 am	✓✓	90	✓			✓	Urgency – damp
12 am	✓	120		Orange	200		
1 pm	✓	140					
2 pm	✓	60					
3 pm	✓	150		Tea	200		
4 pm	✓	100	✓				damp
5 pm	✓	80					
6 pm							
7 pm	✓	150	✓	Beer	500	✓	Urgency – soaked
8 pm							
9 pm							
10 pm	✓	120		Water	100		
11 pm							
12 pm							
1 am							
2 am							
3 am							
4 am							
5 am							
Totals	16	1,520	5		1,750	3	

Please bring your completed diary with you to your next appointment

OBJECTIVE ASSESSMENT

The objective assessment is an assessment of the patient's condition based on what the therapist observes and palpates. A Male Continence Assessment Form is given in the Appendix.

The patient should be given the opportunity to be chaperoned either by a partner or friend, or by a member of staff. The objective assessment should always begin with an explanation of the reason why a digital anal examination is needed. It should be explained that it is necessary to know whether the muscles, which can control continence, are working correctly. The strength of these muscles can be graded (0–6) and the endurance monitored by palpating them. The correct pelvic floor muscle training programme can then be given. The skin sensation and skin condition can also be checked. If the patient declines a digital anal examination, he may allow a perineal examination but he should not be persuaded against his wishes. Following this detailed explanation, the patient must give informed consent to the objective examination and the consent must be entered in the patient notes. At this stage he should be given the opportunity to visit the toilet. For the objective examination, the patient should be lying on his back with two pillows under his head, with his knees bent and his feet on the plinth, without his underwear but with a paper sheet over his pelvis. He may retain his sheath and drainage system if he has one.

ABDOMINAL EXAMINATION

In the supine lying position the abdomen is palpated for pain, pelvic masses and bladder distension. Abdominal examination requires training and practice under medical supervision. Any abnormalities require referral to a GP or urologist.

The ultrasound bladder scan can be performed in this position.

PERINEAL EXAMINATION

The pelvic area may be observed in the supine lying position with knees bent and feet on the bed. The skin condition should be examined for redness, rashes, infection and excoriation in the penile, perineal, scrotal and anal areas. Congenital abnormalities should be noted, such as hypospadias, epispadias or enlarged testis; warts, haemorrhoids or tumours should be noted. All evidence should be recorded.

The patient may then be asked to tighten the anus as if to prevent wind escaping whilst the anal wink is observed. Then he can be asked to tighten at the front as if to prevent the flow of urine and feel a testicular lift and the base of the penis retract into his abdomen. Following which, he is asked to give an unguarded cough which may provide evidence of leakage. He is then requested to cough whilst he is tightening his pelvic floor muscles to prevent leakage which may or may not provide evidence of urinary control.

The fourth sacral (S4) dermatome may be tested using a cotton wool bud or a gloved finger and gently stroking either side of the anus and either side of the perineum whilst asking the patient to describe what he feels. If there is neurological deficit, S2 dermatome may be checked on the lateral surface of the buttock, lateral thigh, posterior calf and plantar heel and S3 dermatome may be checked on the upper two-thirds of the inner surface of the thigh (Figure 3.8). The knee jerk, ankle jerk and plantar reflexes should be tested if neurological impairment is suspected. If there is neurological impairment, the bulbocavernosus reflex test may be performed. The patient should be pre-warned. Using gloves, the therapist exerts gentle pressure on the glans penis with the thumb and index finger during a digital anal examination. If the bulbocavernosus reflex test does not elicit an anal sphincter contraction, there is neurological impairment.

DIGITAL ANAL EXAMINATION

The patient is positioned in supine lying with knees bent and feet on the couch and a paper towel over his abdomen. The therapist approximates a gloved index finger covered amply with lubricating gel to the anal meatus allowing the patient to feel the gel. The patient is then asked to bear down as if he is letting wind escape. Whilst the patient is bearing down, the finger is inserted straight, in a cephalad direction (towards the head) with the finger pad towards the coccyx. The finger can then be introduced to 1–2 cm from the meatus in order to assess the integrity and tone of the external anal sphincter. Any areas of pain should be noted. With a lax sphincter, it may be possible to feel areas of scar tissue in the external anal sphincter where there is no muscle contraction. The patient should be asked to contract the anus and hold for 5 seconds, whilst the therapist grades the strength of the contraction and notes the duration of the hold in seconds. This can be repeated and then the ability to perform a fast contraction noted. Whilst the patient is relaxing, the examining finger is introduced to 3–4 cm from the meatus and the anterior pull of puborectalis gently felt at the anorectal angle. This muscle is then graded, as for any voluntary muscle in the body, 0–6 for muscle strength, for the duration of the hold and for the ability to perform a fast contraction. From this digital anal examination, the anal sphincter and the puborectalis can then be assessed and recorded using the modified Oxford scale (Table 8.3).

URODYNAMICS

Urodynamic investigations study the bladder pressure during filling and voiding, its capacity and flow rate. Cystometric measurements are plotted on a graph or cystometrogram. Patients first sit on a commode over a uroflowmeter to measure the urinary flow rate (Figures 5.1, 8.1 and 8.2). After voiding, two catheters are introduced into the bladder, one to fill the bladder and one attached to a pressure sensor to monitor bladder pressure. A third catheter with a pressure sensor is introduced into the rectum to

Table 8.3. Assessment of male pelvic floor muscle strength

Description	Grade	
Nil	0	No muscle contraction
Flicker	1	Muscle flickers
Weak	2	Weak contraction with no movement
Moderate	3	Moderate contraction with movement
Good	4	Good contraction against resistance
Strong	5	Strong contraction against strong resistance
Very strong	6	Very strong squeeze gripping finger tightly

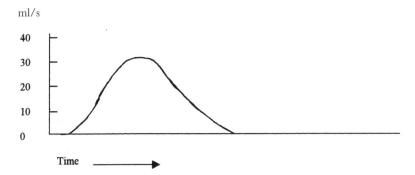

Figure 8.1. Normal flow curve (Reproduced by permission of John Wiley & Sons. *Source*: Dorey, 2001b)

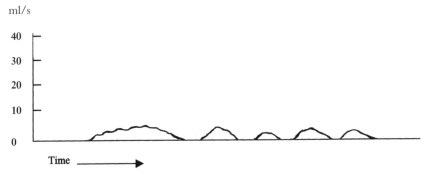

Figure 8.2. Reduced flow due to obstruction or poor bladder contraction (Reproduced by permission of John Wiley & Sons. *Source*: Dorey, 2001b)

measure the intra-abdominal pressure. The pressure of the detrusor muscle is calculated by subtracting the rectal pressure from the intravesical bladder pressure.

detrusor muscle pressure = bladder pressure – abdominal pressure

The bladder is filled with saline or a similar filling medium at room temperature whilst the patient is asked to indicate his first desire to void. He is asked to 'hold on' unless he feels undue discomfort. He may be asked to cough or stand up or walk on the spot in order to provoke evidence. A bladder contraction and leakage of urine demonstrates detrusor overactivity whereas leakage of urine on activity with no bladder contraction demonstrates urodynamic stress urinary incontinence. He is asked to report when he experiences a strong desire to void and when he cannot hold on, then he is asked to void over the flowmeter once more.

A normal bladder will allow filling until the maximum capacity of 400–600 ml is reached. The rise in detrusor pressure should be minimal as the normal bladder stretches to accommodate the filling medium.

Figure 8.3 shows a normal cystometrogram trace, while Figure 8.4 shows the cystometrogram trace of a man with detrusor overactivity. Note the sharp increase in bladder pressure provoked by a cough.

Figure 8.5 shows the cystometrogram trace of a man with stress urinary incontinence. Note the detrusor pressure does not rise with coughing.

Videourodynamics with contrast medium allows visualisation of the bladder, bladder neck and urethra. Ambulatory urodynamics is also utilised in some centres.

Chaudry et al. (1997) stated that many men with apparent lower urinary tract obstruction would have had inappropriate treatment if their manage-

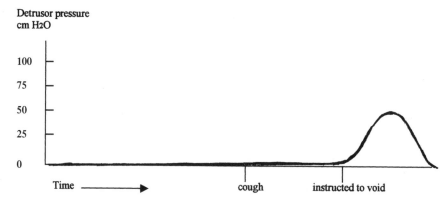

Figure 8.3. Normal cystometrogram trace (Reproduced by permission of John Wiley & Sons. *Source*: Dorey, 2001b)

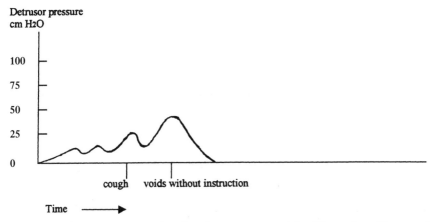

Figure 8.4. Cystometrogram showing detrusor overactivity (Reproduced by permission of John Wiley & Sons. *Source*: Dorey, 2001b)

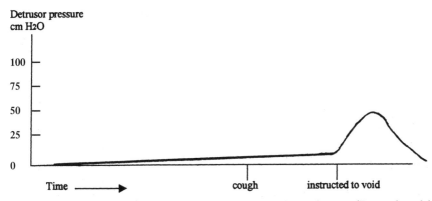

Figure 8.5. Cystometrogram showing stress urinary incontinence (Reproduced by permission of John Wiley & Sons. *Source*: Dorey, 2001b)

ment relied solely on symptom scoring, flow rate and residual urine measurement. They stated that urodynamics should be used in order to provide a predictable subjective and objective outcome of treatment after prostatectomy. Urodynamic findings may not be comparable with history-taking. Vereecken and Wouters (1988) found that there was discrepancy in about a third of cases. They considered that this may be due either to poor history-taking or to the artificial conditions of the examination. Ambulatory urodynamics may provide a better understanding of bladder dysfunction but there were still pitfalls in the presence of artefacts (irregular readings) and the incidence of catheter expulsion during micturition.

SUMMARY

A detailed subjective and objective assessment is necessary in order to make a diagnosis. A digital anal assessment will reveal the strength and endurance of the pelvic floor muscles. A bladder diary provides added information. Urodynamic investigations study the bladder pressure during filling and voiding, its capacity and flow rate.

9 Conservative Treatment

Key points

- Frequency, nocturia, urgency, urge urinary incontinence, stress urinary incontinence, post-micturition dribble can be treated conservatively.
- Treatment progression is patient-specific and dependent on ongoing assessment.
- Treatment modalities include pelvic floor muscle training, biofeedback, electrical stimulation, urge suppression techniques, behavioural modification and advice.

CONSERVATIVE TREATMENT FOR MEN WITH LOWER URINARY TRACT SYMPTOMS

Pelvic floor muscle exercises, biofeedback, electrical stimulation, urge suppression techniques, behavioural modification and advice have all been utilised for the treatment of men with lower urinary tract symptoms (Dorey 2000). Most randomised controlled trials have described the effects of physical therapy for men following prostatectomy (Chapter 10). No randomised controlled trials have reported physiotherapy for urge urinary incontinence. Two randomised controlled trials have supported the intervention of physiotherapy treatment for men with post-micturition dribble (Paterson et al. 1997; Dorey et al. 2004b). Conservative physiotherapy for men with urinary incontinence has evolved from non-randomised and non-controlled trials (Moore & Dorey 1999) in addition to the evidence from randomised controlled trials (Table 9.1).

PATIENT EDUCATION

Most men know little about the prostate gland or its anatomical location. Many are lacking knowledge of any potential medical problems or the treatments available (Smith 1997). In a controlled clinical trial of urinary incontinence, a telephone interview involving 1,140 participants aged 65 years and older in Massachusetts, USA, Branch et al. (1994) found that there were substantial gaps in the knowledge of older persons about urinary incontinence, especially among men aged 85 years and older and those with lower education levels.

Table 9.1. Physiotherapy treatment for urinary incontinence in men

Classification	Symptoms	Treatment options
Urge urinary incontinence	Involuntary leakage of urine accompanied by or immediately preceded by urgency	Urge-suppression techniques Lifestyle modifications Pelvic floor muscle exercises Biofeedback Electrical stimulation (Anticholinergic medication)
Stress urinary incontinence	Involuntary leakage of urine on effort or exertion, or on sneezing or coughing	Pelvic floor muscle exercises 'The knack' Slight pelvic floor muscle contraction while walking Biofeedback Electrical stimulation
Mixed urinary incontinence	Urge urinary incontinence and stress urinary incontinence symptoms	Combination of the above
Post-micturition dribble	Involuntary loss of urine immediately after he has finished passing urine, usually after leaving the toilet	Pelvic floor muscle exercises Strong post-void pelvic floor muscle contraction
Post-prostatectomy incontinence	Stress urinary incontinence symptoms Urge urinary incontinence symptoms Post-micturition dribble	Pre-operative pelvic floor muscle exercises Postoperative pelvic floor muscle exercises Treat as stress urinary incontinence or urge urinary incontinence according to the symptoms Postoperative scar tissue massage
Chronic retention of urine	Non-painful bladder, which remains palpable or percussible after the patient has passed urine. Such patients may be incontinent	Intermittent self-catheterisation (Relief of obstruction)
Functional incontinence	Loss of urine due to functional problems such as poor mobility, difficult clothing or confusion exacerbating existing bladder problems	Improve environment Social care Lifestyle adaptations Clothing adaptations Continence aids

All members of the healthcare team have a responsibility to impart health education in the form of verbal instruction, booklets, diagrams or videos to help people make informed decisions about their lifestyle and health (Edmonds 1991). In a study by the Royal Commission of the NHS as far back as 1978, 95 % of 500 patients questioned found that written information was beneficial and helped to dispel anxiety. Reading matter should have simple terminology and large print.

All treatment should commence with an explanation of the patient's condition and the treatment options available. It is helpful to use the model of the male pelvis complete with musculature in order to explain the basic anatomy and physiology.

STRESS URINARY INCONTINENCE

Stress urinary incontinence in men may occur due to sphincter damage following a prostatectomy (Donnellan et al. 1997). The internal sphincter is damaged in all forms of prostatectomy. Physiotherapy has the potential to be effective in alleviating the stress urinary incontinence caused by an incompetent urethral sphincter by the use of pelvic floor muscle exercises (Van Kampen et al. 2000).

PELVIC FLOOR MUSCLE EXERCISES

The passive urethral mucosal seal is compressed actively by the external urethral sphincter and pelvic floor muscles (Harrison & Abrams 1994). Pelvic floor muscle exercises (PFMEs) are non-invasive and are not associated with serious complications and may be appropriate for patients with stress urinary incontinence who wish to avoid surgery (Gray 1992). Pelvic floor exercises should be individually taught to make sure the patient is lifting up the pelvic floor and not bearing down as if defaecating (i.e. performing a valsalva manoeuvre). The amount and progression of patient-specific pelvic floor exercise is determined by individual assessment and digital anal examination. Men can be encouraged to tighten and lift the pelvic floor muscles strongly as in the control of flatus or the prevention of urine flow. They can practise in front of a mirror to observe a slight retraction of the penis into the body and a testicular lift. Patients can be taught to palpate a contraction of the ischiocavernosus muscle at the perineum 2 cm medially and 2 cm anteriorly to the ischial tuberosity (Figure 9.1).

The convenient positions for practising pelvic floor muscle exercises are in supine lying with knees bent and apart; standing with feet apart; and sitting with knees apart (Van Kampen et al. 2000). It is the intensity rather than frequency of work that is important as maximal voluntary effort causes muscle hypertrophy and increased muscle strength (Dinubile 1991;

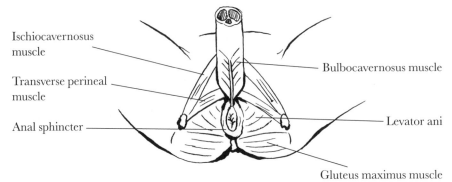

Ischiocavernosus
muscle

Transverse perineal
muscle

Anal sphincter

Bulbocavernosus muscle

Levator ani

Gluteus maximus muscle

Figure 9.1. Male superficial pelvic floor muscles (Reproduced by permission of John Wiley & Sons. *Source*: Dorey, 2001b)

Guyton 1986). In order to achieve full fitness, pelvic floor muscle exercises should be taught for endurance as well as for muscle strength by submaximal contractions (Guyton 1986). Muscle training, therefore, depends on the motivation of the patient and the adherence to the pelvic floor exercise regimen (Jackson et al. 1996). It may help patients to keep an exercise diary.

PELVIC FLOOR MUSCLE STRENGTH

Muscle strength development is achieved by the combination of the recruitment of a greater number of motor units, a higher frequency of excitation and muscle hypertrophy. With increasing load, the recruitment of additional and increasingly larger motor units takes place. When additional force is demanded, both slow and fast twitch fibres are recruited. The intensity rather than the frequency of work is important and high tension must be created to increase strength. Guyton (1986) stated that muscle strength was increased by maximal voluntary effort, which caused muscle hypertrophy. A contraction as close to maximum as possible is required to create high tension in order to address the principles of overload and specificity (Dinubile 1991). There is controversy over the outcomes of increased muscle strength. In one trial pelvic floor muscle strength did not predict the outcome following radical prostatectomy (Jackson et al. 1996). This may have been because the outcome was measured by digital anal assessment. Haslam et al. (1998) found in women that inter-tester reliability could not be assured unless appropriate training was provided. Jackson et al. (1996) used a limited scale, which graded from 0 (no palpable contraction) to 3 (strong), and failed to record the range of muscle strength grades 0 to 6 which are more generally used (Table 8.3).

As with any voluntary muscle training, a weak muscle is strengthened to perform the required task. This means attaining and then maintaining a level of fitness. McArdle et al. (1991) defined fitness as a set of attributes that relate to the ability to perform physical activity. The components of fitness were found to be stamina, suppleness, strength, speed, skill, specificity and spirit, as shown in Table 9.2 (Norris 2004).

Table 9.2. Components of fitness ('S' factors)
(Reproduced by permission of Elsevier. *Source*:
Norris, 2000)

Stamina
Suppleness
Strength
Speed
Skill
Specificity
Spirit

PELVIC FLOOR MUSCLE ENDURANCE

In order to achieve full fitness, pelvic floor muscle exercises should be taught for endurance as well as for muscle strength. Guyton (1986) stated that endurance is the time limit of a person's ability to maintain either a static (isometric) force or a power level of dynamic exercise. He also found that endurance was improved by submaximal repetitive contractions. Both static and dynamic endurance are necessary for normal pelvic floor performance. Static endurance is defined as the interval in which a maximal or submaximal contraction can be maintained, whereas dynamic endurance is the number of contractions performed with constant frequency and load before exhaustion takes place (Christensen & Fuglsang-Frederiksen 1998).

'THE KNACK'

'The knack' is the ability to initiate a pelvic floor muscle contraction sufficiently far in advance of an intra-abdominal pressure rise (Miller et al. 1996). It is called 'the knack' in recognition of the motor control skill required. There is controversy about the voluntary control and innervation of the urinary sphincter. It may be that it contracts with the pelvic floor muscles but this action has not been identified. The key to bladder control may be in the urethral sphincter 'guarding reflex' identified in cats (Garry et al. 1959). In 1997, Park et al. revisited the guarding reflex and stated that pelvic floor exercises may affect continence by increasing the ability to 'guard' or contract quickly during times of increased intra-abdominal pressure. Gordon and Logue (1985) found that the upright position when standing and walking stimulated the pelvic floor reflex and Mahony et al. (1977) stated that increased pelvic floor tone should diminish nocturia.

SPECIFIC HOME EXERCISE PROGRAMME

There has been no research conducted to give clear indications of the number of pelvic floor muscle exercises to perform in order to build up muscle bulk, strength and endurance. Kegel (1956) instructed female patients to exercise the pelvic floor muscles two or three times a day for 20 minutes using a perineometer. In addition patients performed pelvic floor muscle exercises 5 to 10 times every half hour during the day. This amounted to about 300 contractions a day. In muscle building, it is the quality not the quantity that is important. Research has shown that a few maximal home exercises twice a day in lying, sitting and standing were effective in increasing pelvic floor muscle strength (Dorey et al. 2004a). Randomised controlled trials are needed to ascertain the number of repetitions needed to gain optimum relief of symptoms. It may be that exercises do not need to be performed every day. When men are given pelvic floor muscle exercises to perform every hour, they will feel guilty if they are unable to comply. Many therapists give patients more exercises than they need in the hope of getting a degree of compliance. In order to gain compliance, it is surely better to have an honest agreement with the patient and let him know the exact number of contractions required.

MOTIVATION AND COMPLIANCE

Muscle training depends on the motivation of the patient and the adherence to the pelvic floor exercise regimen (Jackson et al. 1996). Knight and Laycock (1994) stated that the success of pelvic floor muscle exercises depended on a high level of patient motivation and compliance in women. Wilson et al. (2002) concluded that female patients performed pelvic floor muscle exercises better when they attended outpatient departments and were less motivated when left to a scheme of home exercises. However, Holley et al. (1995) found that only 1 out of 10 women suffering from urodynamic stress urinary incontinence were sufficiently motivated to perform pelvic floor muscle exercises after 5 years.

PELVIC FLOOR MUSCLE EXERCISES FOR STRESS URINARY INCONTINENCE

Pelvic floor muscle exercises should be patient-specific. The hold time in seconds is ascertained from the digital anal assessment. The rest time should exceed the hold time to allow muscle fibre recovery. There is no evidence for an optimum number of repeat contractions; however, the objective assessment will help determine what is appropriate for each patient. The quality of contraction is more important than the quantity. Exercises should be practised every day and include some fast and some slow contractions. A typical programme practised twice a day could be: three maximal contractions in supine lying with knees bent, three maximal contractions in sitting and three maximal contractions in standing, held for the length of time in seconds specific to the patient. However, this is only a guide. Some contractions may be activated quickly and some slowly. The patient can also be encouraged to lift the pelvic floor up 50 % of their maximum whilst walking to encourage postural support. Men can be taught 'the knack' of tightening the pelvic floor muscles before and during activities which increase the intra-abdominal pressure, such as coughing, sneezing, rising from sitting or lifting (Ashton-Miller & DeLancey 1996).

BIOFEEDBACK TREATMENT FOR STRESS INCONTINENCE

Biofeedback is the technique by which information about a normally unconscious physiological process is presented to the patient and/or the therapist as a visual, auditory or tactile signal (Abrams et al. 2002). Biofeedback is a mechanism by which the patient is made more aware of pelvic floor muscle activity and is encouraged to greater muscular effort (Van Kampen et al. 2000). Many patients are unable to contract their pelvic floor or do not understand the maximal effort needed. Biofeedback can often provide the necessary awareness for muscle re-education. There are three recognised methods of biofeedback: digital, manometric (pressure) and electromyographic. The three biofeedback methods have been studied and compared vaginally and they appeared to be well correlated with one another in women (Haslam 1999).

Digital anal biofeedback

A lubricated, gloved index finger can be used during a digital anal examination to monitor the strength and endurance of the external anal sphincter and the puborectalis muscle (Chapter 8). The information can then be communicated to the patient in order to provide feedback and encouragement.

Manometric biofeedback

An anal pressure probe can be used to monitor muscle activity and provide manometric (pressure) biofeedback. Anal manometry is a reliable method of monitoring pelvic floor muscle strength when performed by one operator (Dorey & Swinkels 2003). The anal balloon probe may be attached to a perineometer with a visual display (Figure 9.2). Sophisticated computerised equipment with a coloured visual display screen, audible feedback, a variety of work and rest programmes, and a printer is considered the gold standard by many

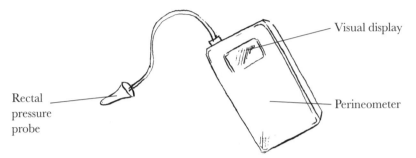

Visual display

Rectal
pressure
probe

Perineometer

Figure 9.2. Perineometer with anal pressure probe (Reproduced by permission of John Wiley & Sons. *Source*: Dorey, 2001b)

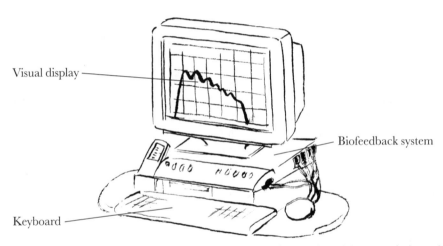

Visual display

Biofeedback system

Keyboard

Figure 9.3. Computerised biofeedback equipment (Reproduced by permission of John Wiley & Sons. *Source*: Dorey, 2001b)

therapists (Figure 9.3). This equipment may be used for manometry, EMG and electrical stimulation. The patient should be placed in supine lying with his knees bent and apart with a paper sheet over his pelvis. He should be able to see and hear the monitor screen. The anal pressure probe should be covered with a condom, lubricated with gel and approximated to the patient's anus (Figure 9.4). The patient is then asked to bear down as if releasing flatus whilst the probe is gently inserted. The probe needs to be held in position to record maximal readings and to prevent the probe from slipping out. The difficulty with an anal pressure probe is that it records the activity of both the anal sphincter and the puborectalis muscle. It is important to record the activity of the puborectalis muscle, which lies above and is integrated with the pubococcygeus muscle which surrounds the external urethral sphincter.

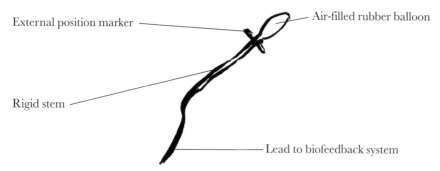

External position marker

Air-filled rubber balloon

Rigid stem

Lead to biofeedback system

Figure 9.4. Anal pressure probe (Reproduced by permission of John Wiley & Sons. *Source*: Dorey, 2001b)

The pressure is usually measured in bars or numerical units on a perineometer or by centimetres of water (cm H_2O) or millimetres of mercury (mm Hg) on more accurate manometric equipment.

Small portable pressure biofeedback units can be used with an anal pressure probe for home use.

Electromyographic biofeedback

Electromyography (EMG) is the study of minute electrical potentials produced by depolarisation of the muscle membrane (Siroky 1996). Bioelectric activity of the muscles can be recorded using either a needle sensor, an anal probe or surface sensors. The bioelectric activity is measured in units of microvolts (μV).

Needle EMG, which is invasive and may be painful, is currently out of the scope of nurses and physiotherapists.

The *anal EMG probe* is strictly for single patient use. It is applied using lubricating gel and asking the patient to bear down as if letting wind escape. Most probes need to be held by the therapist to prevent slippage. New, shaped, anal electrodes fit snugly into position and allow ambulatory use (Figure 9.5). The anal probe is attached to a computerised biofeedback machine, which will monitor the bioelectric activity of the muscles by EMG biofeedback and provide a coloured visual display and sometimes an audible signal to encourage greater effort. Small, portable EMG units can be used with an anal probe for home use.

Surface skin sensors may be used on the perineum. They can be used to monitor the activity of the pubococcygeus and the ischiococcygeus muscles. The skin needs to be cleansed with an alcohol swab to remove any oils that may prevent a good contact. It may be necessary to shave the area. New surface sensors should be used for each treatment. Two small sticky surface sensors may be placed longitudinally over the pubococcygeus and the ischio-coccygeus muscle to be monitored by EMG and may be placed 1 cm lateral to the midline (Figure 9.6). A third sensor may be placed over a bony point such as the sacrum or coccyx to act as a reference (grounding) to cut out extraneous 'noise' from the electrical activity of other muscles in the area. However, some EMG equipment uses a triangular arrangement for all three sensors with the two active sensors longitudinal to the muscle fibres. One of the benefits of EMG is its use in functional positions. Problems associated with the use of EMG may be due to the size of the sensor pad or probe which may pick up electrical activity from the surrounding muscles. However, surface EMG is non-invasive and painless, and can also be used as an initiator of cerebral control, a tool of assessment, a motivator and a method of record-ing; it can be used to both encourage and challenge the patient (Haslam 1998) (Figure 9.7).

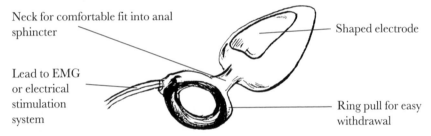

Figure 9.5. Anal probe for EMG or electrical stimulation (Reproduced by permission of John Wiley & Sons. *Source*: Dorey, 2001b)

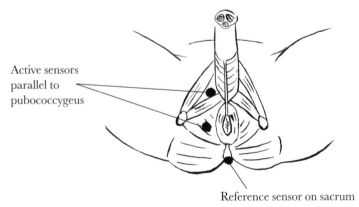

Figure 9.6. Position of surface sensors for EMG biofeedback (Reproduced by permission of John Wiley & Sons. *Source*: Dorey, 2001b)

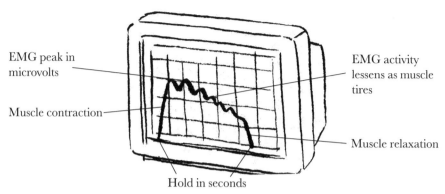

EMG peak in microvolts

EMG activity lessens as muscle tires

Muscle contraction

Muscle relaxation

Hold in seconds

Figure 9.7. EMG biofeedback shown on a computer screen (Reproduced by permission of John Wiley & Sons. *Source*: Dorey, 2001b)

ELECTRICAL STIMULATION FOR STRESS INCONTINENCE

There are two basic types of electrical stimulation which have been used on pelvic floor muscles: maximal electrical stimulation and low-intensity electrical stimulation.

Maximal electrical stimulation is applied pulsed at the maximum intensity tolerable for short periods of 20 minutes at a frequency of about 30 Hz to produce a tetanic contraction and is used for stress urinary incontinence.

Low-intensity electrical stimulation may be applied pulsed or continuous for several hours a day for several months. However, continuous low-intensity electrical stimulation can lead to a conversion of muscle fibre type from fast-twitch (type 2) to slow-twitch (type 1) (Salmons & Henriksonn 1981). This may produce an undesired effect as the recruitment of fast-twitch fibres of the pelvic floor muscles are necessary during rises in intra-abdominal pressure.

Electrical stimulation of the pelvic floor muscles may be delivered by anal or surface electrodes. The anal electrode contains positive and negative bands and is used alone. It is strictly for single patient use. Surface electrodes may be placed on the coccyx and the perineum or on either side of the perineal body as shown in Figure 9.8. Care should be taken to avoid burning that may occur with small electrodes. Skin sensation should be tested before treatment and the skin should be viewed after treatment. Contraindications for electrical stimulation are listed in Table 9.3.

A current of sufficient amplitude will excite nerve and muscle tissue in its field causing a muscular contraction. Electrical stimulation has been used for patients who are initially unable to contract their pelvic floor muscles. However, Berghmans et al. (1998) noted that in five randomised controlled trials (RCTs) in women, electrical stimulation was found to be no more effective than PFMEs alone. In fact, Knight and Laycock (1998) found that pulsed

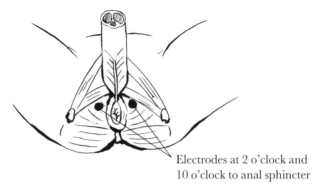

Electrodes at 2 o'clock and
10 o'clock to anal sphincter

Figure 9.8. Position of surface electrodes for electrical stimulation (Reproduced by permission of John Wiley & Sons. *Source*: Dorey, 2001b)

Table 9.3. Contraindications for electrical stimulation

Lack of consent
Patient is anxious
Patient lacks understanding
Broken skin in the area
Metal in the field (will concentrate the current and lead to a burn)
Patients with severe cardiac problems
Patients with pacemakers
Cancer
Loss of sensation
Poor circulation
Epilepsy
Recent surgery
Recent or recurrent haemorrhages

low-intensity electrical stimulation may have a detrimental influence on female patients with urodynamic stress urinary incontinence. In men, even less research has been conducted.

The real clinical benefit of electrical stimulation remains to be clarified. It may be that it can increase the circulation to the pelvic floor or it may be useful to show patients how to initially contract the pelvic floor muscles.

In men, electrical stimulation has been used for stress urinary incontinence at a frequency of 30 to 50 Hz. This wavelength produces a tetanic contraction with minimal risk of undue muscle fatigue, provided that the pulse train off-time is equal to or exceeds the on-time. Knight and Laycock (1994) stated that a pulse width of 200 microseconds produced excitation at relatively low current intensity and was more comfortable than shorter pulse widths. They suggested that acute maximal electrical stimulation may benefit patients with very weak pelvic floor muscles.

Electrical stimulation has been used for men with stress urinary incontinence post-prostatectomy (Bennett et al. 1997; Hirakawa et al. 1993; Kraus & Lilien 1981; Moore et al. 1999; Sotiropoulos et al. 1976). However, the treatment has been combined with pelvic floor muscle exercises in two studies (Hirakawa et al. 1993; Moore et al. 1999) and the sample size in each case was small. In the only two randomised controlled trials, Bennett et al. (1997) and Moore et al. (1999) both found no improvement compared to control groups.

URGE URINARY INCONTINENCE

The storage symptoms of frequency, nocturia, urgency and urge urinary incontinence can be treated with pelvic floor muscle exercises, urge-suppression techniques, and behavioural modifications including fluid intake advice (Burgio et al. 1989; Dorey 1998; Van Kampen et al. 2000).

PELVIC FLOOR MUSCLE EXERCISES FOR URGE
URINARY INCONTINENCE

Pelvic floor muscle exercises can be used for urge urinary incontinence to strengthen the pelvic floor musculature and regain the ability to control the urge to void urine. It is suggested that when the pelvic floor contracts the detrusor muscle will relax due to the activity of the perineopudendal facilitative reflex (Mahony et al. 1977) (Chapter 4). Muscle training can be enhanced by the use of biofeedback as discussed in the treatment for stress urinary incontinence.

ELECTRICAL STIMULATION FOR URGE
URINARY INCONTINENCE

Urge urinary incontinence may be treated with continuous biphasic electrical stimulation at a frequency of 5–10 Hz with a pulse width of 200 microseconds for up to 20 minutes for urge suppression (Fall & Lindstrom 1991; Jones 1994). Geirsson and Fall (1997) used stimulation parameters of 0.75 milliseconds with continuous biphasic waves and a frequency of 5 Hz in the treatment of detrusor overactivity in order to cause reflex inhibition of detrusor contractions. Some units provide intermittent biphasic electrical stimulation at 5–10 Hz for urge urinary incontinence.

LIFESTYLE CHANGES AND BEHAVIOURAL MODIFICATIONS
FOR URGE URINARY INCONTINENCE

There are several non-invasive techniques which singly or combined may improve the symptoms of frequency, nocturia, urgency and urge urinary incontinence. These include urge suppression, treating constipation, weight reduction, the adjustment of fluids, and the review of medications including diuretics. In collaboration with other members of the healthcare team, bowel management, weight loss, medication review and treatment of urinary tract infection may all improve symptoms. Education, attention to quantity, type and timing of fluid intake, avoiding constipation and suppressing the urge to micturate are now considered part of lifestyle changes which can alter previous behaviour patterns. Owing to the limitations of the latest research, current knowledge and practice is based on opinion and consensus but not on strong evidence.

URGE SUPPRESSION FOR URGE URINARY INCONTINENCE

Bladder training (Frewen 1979), also termed bladder retraining (Mahady & Begg 1981), bladder drill (Elder & Stephenson 1980), bladder re-education (Millard & Oldenburg 1983) and urge suppression, is a method of consciously suppressing the urge to void in order to delay micturition and increase functional bladder capacity (Wells 1988). Frewen (1979) emphasised the psychological aspects of detrusor overactivity, which may be influenced by life events. Urge-suppression techniques include strategies such as keeping calm, sitting down or standing still and waiting one minute until the urge disappears. Once the urge has abated, men can either walk calmly to the bathroom or continue their activities, thus allowing their bladder to stretch and fill further (see Table 9.4). If men rush to the toilet mid-urge, they may leak urine. Patients undergoing urge suppression need considerable encouragement, motivation and determination to succeed.

FLUID INTAKE

Guyton (1986) stated that normal fluid intake averages 2,300 ml per day of which two-thirds (1,518 ml) is direct fluid and the remaining third is a product of food synthesis. Weisberg (1982) found a helpful gauge was 14 ml to 20 ml of fluid intake per pound of body weight. It may be more helpful to monitor the 24-hour urine output, which should be about 1,000 to 1,500 ml. Normal

Table 9.4. Urge-suppression techniques

Keep calm
Stand still or sit down
Relax the abdominal muscles
Wait for 1 minute until the urge disappears
When the urge has disappeared visit the toilet or continue previous activities
Never rush to the toilet mid-urge

intake should be increased during hot weather, with strenuous activity and when eating salty foods. No-one should ever be thirsty. If the urine is dark, the patient should be encouraged to drink more fluid. However, some food products, vitamins and medication can affect the colour of urine (Chapter 12). Water is the best fluid to drink.

Moul (1998) listed foods and beverages which may irritate the bladder and may lead to detrusor overactivity. These foods included citrus products, tomato products, highly spiced foods, sugar, honey, chocolate and corn syrup, whilst the beverages included alcohol, colas, milk, coffee, tea, and other drinks containing caffeine. Anecdotal reports suggest that caffeine reduction relieves symptoms in people with detrusor overactivity. Randomised controlled trials are needed to confirm the effect these products have on the bladder.

DIURETICS

Natural diuretics are commonly xanthines, such as caffeine and theobromine, occurring primarily in beverages, which act chemically in the body to increase urine production. Caffeine occurs naturally in about 60 species of plants, most commonly coffee beans, tea leaves, cocoa seeds and the cola nut (Moore 1990). Caffeine is also added to several over-the-counter medicines, to counteract the drowsiness that the side-effect of the drug produces or to enhance analgesic absorption (Wells 1988). Caffeine is a bladder irritant and stimulant with a diuretic effect. It also lowers urethral pressure (Palermo & Zimskind 1977). It can cause the smooth muscle of the detrusor to contract with implications of nocturia, frequency, urgency and urge urinary incontinence (Addison 1997). Addison (1997) considered that men who are particularly at risk are those with detrusor overactivity, neurological disease and the elderly. However, he stated caffeine should be reduced slowly over a 3-week period in order to prevent withdrawal symptoms of headaches or drowsiness.

CRANBERRY JUICE

In the nineteenth century, the North American Indians used crushed cranberries as a herbal remedy for the treatment of urinary tract infections (Bodel et al. 1959; Moen 1962). Although many studies have focused on the alteration in urinary pH (Fellers et al. 1933) or the increased hippuric acid levels (Bodel et al. 1959; Kinney & Blount 1979), it is also believed that cranberry juice has a bacteriostatic effect by affecting the adherence of certain organisms, in particular *Escherichia coli*, to the lining of the bladder (Beachy 1981).

Avorn et al. (1994) conducted a randomised controlled trial with a sample of elderly women consuming either 300ml of cranberry juice or a placebo. Results showed that cranberry juice reduced the occurrence of bacteriuria with pyuria.

Addison (1997) recommended cranberry juice for those patients with a high risk of urinary tract infection, those with cystitis from *Escherichia coli*, patients with indwelling catheters, those undertaking intermittent self-catheterisation or those using sheath drainage. He considered that the recommendation of cranberry juice should be supported by written patient information and be monitored and recorded with dosage, patient instructions, contraindications, side-effects and expected outcomes. Drinking in excess of 1 litre of cranberry juice a day over a prolonged period may increase the risk of uric stone formation (Rogers 1991). Other side-effects include gastritis and, for rheumatoid arthritis sufferers, increased joint pain (Addison 1997) and, in patients with irritable bowel syndrome, diarrhoea (Leaver 1996). Diabetics could find an increase in blood sugar level. For patients who simply do not like the taste, or find the juice too expensive, cranberry juice capsules can be purchased in health shops, but there is no research on their effectiveness or comparison with cranberry juice (Leaver 1996). Cranberry juice is contraindicated for patients on warfarin.

SMOKING

Nicotine makes the smooth muscle in the body contract and is linked to detrusor overactivity (Haidinger et al. 2000). A review of the literature showed that smoking was also linked to erectile dysfunction (Dorey 2001a).

MEDICATION FOR URGE URINARY INCONTINENCE

For men with severe urge urinary incontinence and for men with nocturnal enuresis, anticholinergic medication may be helpful whilst they are receiving conservative treatment. The side-effects of anticholinergic medication include a dry mouth, drowsiness, constipation and vision accommodation difficulties (Chapter 12).

ACUPUNCTURE FOR URGE URINARY INCONTINENCE

Acupuncture and electro-acupuncture have been used for urge urinary incontinence. Treatment should be given by a therapist specialised in acupuncture. More research is needed in this area.

POST-PROSTATECTOMY INCONTINENCE

Post-prostatectomy incontinence should be treated according to the presenting symptoms. Usually this is either stress urinary incontinence or urge urinary incontinence but many patients present with a combination of both called mixed incontinence (Chapter 11).

POST-MICTURITION DRIBBLE

Patients suffering from post-micturition dribble have historically used a self-help technique called bulbar urethral massage, or urethral milking, to ease this distressing condition. The patient is taught, after urinating, to place his fingers behind the scrotum and gently massage the bulbar urethra in a forwards and upwards direction in order to 'milk' the remaining urine from the urethra. In a randomised single-blind trial to test the efficacy of urethral milking, Paterson et al. (1997) found pelvic floor muscle exercises to be twice as effective as urethral milking and recommended pelvic floor exercises as a treatment for this condition. Dorey et al. (2004b) found that contracting the pelvic floor muscles strongly after voiding facilitated a contraction of the bulbocavernosus muscle and eliminated urine from the bulbar portion of the urethra while men were still poised over the toilet. Dorey et al. (2004b) reported that this strong post-void contraction replaced the normal post-void reflex bulbocavernosus muscle contraction and superseded bulbar milking. Some men try to bear down to empty the bladder fully to prevent the after-dribble. In fact, men should be taught to tighten their pelvic floor muscles up strongly after voiding urine instead of bearing down.

CHRONIC RETENTION OF URINE

Chronic retention of urine is defined as a non-painful bladder, which remains palpable or percussible after the patient has passed urine (Abrams et al. 2002). Such patients may be incontinent. Catheterisation is a technique for bladder emptying in which a catheter is employed to drain the bladder or a urinary reservoir (Abrams et al. 2002). Intermittent catheterisation is defined as drainage or aspiration of the bladder or a urinary reservoir with subsequent removal of the catheter (Abrams et al. 2002). Clean, intermittent self-catheterisation is used for patients with incomplete emptying due to detrusor underactivity, acontractile detrusor, or detrusor/sphincter dyssynergia. Detrusor underactivity is defined as a contraction of reduced strength and/or duration, resulting in prolonged bladder emptying and/or a failure to achieve complete bladder emptying within a normal time span (Abrams et al. 2002). Acontractile detrusor is one that cannot be demonstrated to contract during urodynamic studies (Abrams et al. 2002). It may occur owing to lack of neurological control or detrusor overstretching. Overstretching may also cause pelvic nerve compression. Detrusor/sphincter dyssynergia is defined as a detrusor contraction concurrent with an involuntary contraction of the urethral and/or periurethral striated muscle (Abrams et al. 2002). Occasionally flow may be prevented altogether. It is due to neurological impairment. Men with neurogenic detrusor overactivity may benefit by clean, intermittent self-catheterisation, a sheath drainage system or, as a last resort, an indwelling catheter. For patients who are permanently catheterised, a suprapubic catheter is more acceptable. Medication, in the form of anticholinergic drugs, or surgery, such as a clam ileocystoplasty, sphincterotomy for detrusor dyssynergia or sacral root stimulation by neuromodulation may be necessary.

INTERMITTENT SELF-CATHETERISATION

Clean, intermittent self-catheterisation is used for men who are unable to completely empty their bladder by normal voiding. Men in this category include spinal injury patients and those with outflow obstruction.

Plastic catheters used for clean, intermittent self-catheterisation fall into three groups:

1. Catheters requiring lubrication prior to insertion.
2. Those with a hydrophilic coating, which when activated by water, provide a lubricated smooth surface for single use.
3. Self-lubricated, silicone-coated catheters for single use.

Other considerations are the position and smoothness of the drainage eyes in order to reduce the risk of urethral trauma. Patient preference will be influenced by convenience, ease of insertion, ease of removal and cost.

ARTIFICIAL URINARY SPHINCTER

A pressure-regulated, artificial urinary sphincter has been developed which overcomes many deficiencies of earlier devices (Craggs et al. 1991). It can be implanted surgically for patients with incontinence who have not responded to conservative treatment. It consists of a cuff round the urethra, a reservoir implanted in the abdomen, and a pump implanted in the scrotum (Figure 9.9). To commence micturition, the scrotal pump is squeezed several times which transfers fluid from the urethral cuff into the abdominal reservoir. The cuff is automatically re-inflated after 2 or 3 minutes. In response to increased intra-abdominal pressure, additional fluid flows into the cuff to give extra intra-urethral pressure. The operation of this device needs good manual dexterity. The associated risks are mechanical failure, rejection and erosion through the urethra often requiring revision (Denning 1996).

CLAM ILEOCYSTOPLASTY

Clam ileocystoplasty is an operation in which a portion of the ileum is used to augment the bladder. This operation is designed to overcome detrusor overactivity. The bladder is opened up like a clam and a portion of ileum with its own blood supply is sewn to the bladder to increase bladder capacity. However, the transplanted ileum continues to produce mucus, which may form

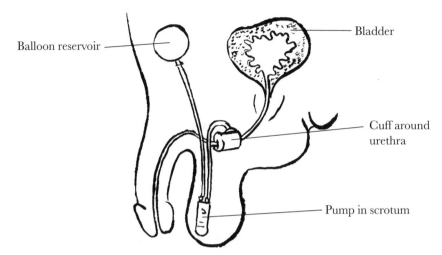

Balloon reservoir

Bladder

Cuff around urethra

Pump in scrotum

Figure 9.9. Artificial urinary sphincter (Reproduced by permission of John Wiley & Sons. *Source*: Dorey, 2001b)

a plug in the urethra causing retention. Some patients have problems emptying the bladder completely and need to use intermittent self-catheterisation.

SACRAL NEUROMODULATION

Electrical stimulation of peripheral nerves can be used to cause muscle contraction, to activate reflexes, and to modulate some functions of the central nervous system (Jezernik et al. 2002). If applied to the spinal cord or nerves controlling the lower urinary tract, electrical stimulation can produce bladder or sphincter contraction, and produce micturition in men with incontinence and urinary retention due to neurological damage and spinal injury. Sacral neuromodulation is performed by surgically implanting an electrode into the third sacral foramina to stimulate the third sacral nerve (S3) in order to maintain continence. The electrode is connected to a stimulator implanted into the abdominal cavity. The device may be turned on to allow bladder filling and off to allow voiding with a magnet held over the stimulator. Post-surgery problems of infection, migration of the electrodes and pain can occur.

EXTRA-URETHRAL URINARY INCONTINENCE

Extra-urethral urinary incontinence occurs when the distal end of the ureter opens into a place other than the bladder such as the rectum or perineum. A fistula or passageway connecting the bladder to the bowel resulting from trauma or infection following surgery will also cause extra-urethral incontinence. Patients with extra-urethral incontinence need to be referred for surgery.

FUNCTIONAL INCONTINENCE

Functional incontinence is incontinence that is caused by problems of mobility and dexterity. It is not included in the International Continence Society classification of incontinence. Men with functional incontinence find it difficult to reach the toilet in time due to physical and environmental factors. Functional incontinence should be treated by improving the patient's environment, by social care and aids, and by lifestyle and clothing adaptations.

FOLLOW-UP TREATMENT

At the end of the treatment session, it is helpful to make a list of questions to ask the patient when he attends for his next treatment. The progression in the number of repetitions and increase in hold time of pelvic floor muscle exercises will depend on the results of another digital anal assessment to ascertain the strength and endurance of the pelvic floor muscles.

TREATMENT OUTCOMES

Treatment aims to achieve urinary control, continence and confidence by conservative measures. However, it is not always possible to gain this outcome and patients may need help with managing their condition. It is important to set realistic goals.

PREVENTION OF URINARY INCONTINENCE

There are no trials concerning preventative pelvic floor exercises for men or women. However, it seems reasonable to suppose that keeping the pelvic floor muscles in good tone would be beneficial in maintaining their normal function.

PADS

All patients should have a full continence assessment before being given pads. Conservative treatment may prevent the need for pads. However, patients may wish to wear a pad for confidence while receiving therapy, and some patients who find no improvement with therapy may wish to manage the problem themselves.

Pads are usually composed of three layers: a non-woven surface, absorbent wood-pulp or tissue paper, and a waterproof backing (Pomfret 1996). The size and shape of pads varies. Men may need the help of continence advisors to select a pad that is comfortable, contains the urine and the odour, and is reasonably priced. Stretch pants may hold the pad in place. Men with post-micturition dribble may wish to use a dribble collector (Figure 9.10). This specially designed pouch has a pocket for the penis and testicles. A specially designed, adhesive backing sticks the collector to the inside of tightly fitting briefs.

In an evaluation of 36 all-in-one disposable, shaped incontinence pads (Figure 9.11), Pettersson and Fader (2000) found that there were wide variations in cost and absorbency and that price was a poor indicator of performance. From 192 recruits from 37 residential nursing homes, participants and carers indicated that a successful product needed to be able to contain urine without leaking and to have tabs for ease of opening and resealing.

The Association for Continence Advice undertook a survey of 1,915 men and women with incontinence for the National Care Audit (ACA Survey

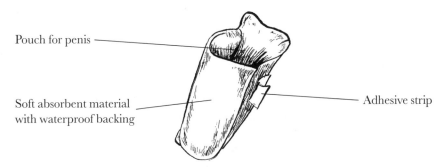

Figure 9.10. Dribble pouch (Reproduced by permission of John Wiley & Sons. *Source*: Dorey, 2001b)

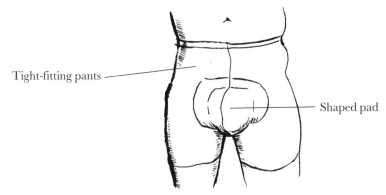

Figure 9.11. Shaped incontinence pad (Reproduced by permission of John Wiley & Sons. *Source*: Dorey, 2001b)

2000). They found that 25 % of men used disposable pads, 6 % of men used re-usable pads, 28 % of men used a sheath and drainage system while only 7 % of men managed their bladder problems with pelvic floor exercises.

APPLIANCES

All patients should have a full continence assessment before being given appliances. The most common appliance is the sheath and leg bag (Figure 9.12). Conservative therapy can be given with the sheath and leg bag in place. Continence advisors are skilled at fitting the correct size of sheath, which allows for changes in penis size. Some sheaths adhere to the penis whilst some have waist bands and groin straps (Pomfret 1996). Skin care is paramount.

PENILE CLAMP

The penile clamp (Figure 9.13) is still being used by some men to control their incontinence. Improperly used, the clamp may cause pressure necrosis to the penis and is therefore not usually recommended as a treatment option.

SKIN CARE

Incontinence dermatitis is caused by a rise in the pH of the skin making it more acid, increased permeability, increased hydration, attack by faecal enzymes, the action of certain skin preparations and the use of urine containment products (Le Lievre 1999). The skin of men with incontinence dermatitis and urinary incontinence should be cared for as shown in Table 9.5.

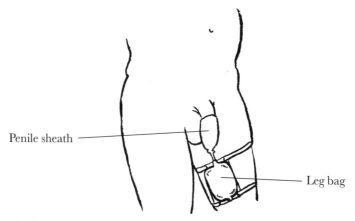

Penile sheath

Leg bag

Figure 9.12. Sheath and leg bag (Reproduced by permission of John Wiley & Sons. *Source*: Dorey, 2001b)

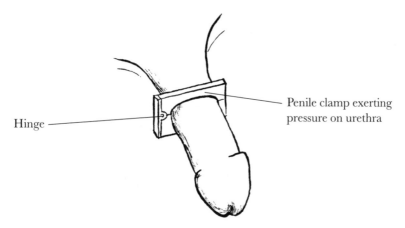

Figure 9.13. Penile clamp (Reproduced by permission of John Wiley & Sons. *Source*: Dorey, 2001b)

Table 9.5. Skin care for incontinent patients (reproduced, with permission, from Dorey (2001b))

Avoid soaps and detergents which wash away protective oils
Wash in warm water alone or minimal amount of mild non-perfumed soap
Avoid high-temperature baths
Avoid soaking in the bath
Avoid talcum powder
Use only creams which contain high quantities of zinc
Pat skin completely dry and avoid vigorous rubbing
Use pads with super-absorbency which separate the urine from the skin
Check for latex allergy for men with sheaths and catheters
Avoid plastic pants and sheets which cause sweating

RESEARCH OPPORTUNITIES

The challenge for professionals will be the integration of clinical evidence into practice and promoting and implementing prevention strategies. More research is needed to supplement these initiatives.

(Consensus Statement 1997)

SUGGESTIONS FOR FUTURE RESEARCH

Further quantitative and qualitative research is needed to explore the benefits of conservative treatment for men with lower urinary tract symptoms. Collaborative multi-centre studies could involve input from urologists, nurses and physiotherapists in order to justify or improve on the current treatment regimes.

Qualitative research in the form of focus groups or in-depth interviews of urologists, nurses, physiotherapists and patients could identify the training needs of physiotherapists and nurses in this field. Specialised training could be provided to improve and extend professional competencies.

Randomised controlled trials could explore the following topics:

- Optimum number, frequency and strength of pelvic floor muscle repetitions for the effective treatment of men with lower urinary tract symptoms.
- Optimum position for performing pelvic floor muscle exercises.
- Use of 'the knack' for men with stress urinary incontinence.
- Optimum time to begin pre-prostatectomy exercises.
- Effectiveness of immediate post-prostatectomy exercises (contracting gently on the catheter).
- Comparison of anal and surface EMG biofeedback in men.
- Type, parameters and intensity of electrical stimulation for stress urinary incontinence and urge urinary incontinence in men.
- Behavioural and lifestyle changes for men with lower urinary tract symptoms.

CASE STUDIES: QUESTIONS AND ANSWERS

(1) A post-prostatectomy patient complains of leakage since his operation.

Q. How would you differentiate between:
   (a) urge urinary incontinence,
   (b) stress urinary incontinence,
   (c) post-micturition dribble, and
   (d) chronic retention of urine?

A. A bladder diary would show the number of voids, the amount voided, the amount of intake and output, the type of fluid drunk and the number of leaks of urine day and night. If there are nine or more voids per 24 hours (normal about seven) and more than three voids at night, the patient may be suffering from frequency, urgency, urge urinary incontinence and nocturia and may develop a low-compliance bladder. From the bladder diary it can be determined whether the patient is drinking excessively (normal intake is from 1,000 to 1,500 ml per day) as a cause of increased frequency. It is useful to monitor the urinary output. Urodynamics is a more invasive way of diagnosing stress urinary incontinence or urge urinary incontinence. The patient should be asked if his stream is reduced or if he is suffering from hesitancy and intermittency in case he has blockage from a stricture. Stress urinary incontinence post-prostatectomy may be described subjectively as uncontrolled spurts of urine during activities which increase the intra-abdominal pressure. Post-micturition dribble is leakage after micturition has been completed and the patient moves away from the bathroom. Post-micturition dribble should be distinguished from terminal dribble which is a dribble at the end of micturition.

(2) A patient complains of increased urgency and frequency for 3 months. He has noticed some blood in his urine.

Q. What are the possible diagnoses?

A. This patient could be suffering from a bladder infection, urethritis or bladder cancer. He would need a urine culture and possible antibiotics. If he has had a recent prostatectomy he may suffer with haematuria. Haematuria is also a sign of bladder cancer. He would need referring to a urologist for a cystoscopy.

(3) A patient complains of increased problems of poor stream and difficulty initiating the stream. Recently he has been suffering from severe urge urinary incontinence.

Q. How would you treat this patient?

A. This patient presents with increasing symptoms of obstruction. In addition he has developed symptoms of detrusor overactivity. He would need referral to a urologist who would perform a digital rectal examination to exclude prostate cancer, and send the patient for uroflowmetry, an ultrasound scan to eliminate retention, and a blood test for prostate-specific antigen (PSA). If the urologist diagnoses benign prostatic hyperplasia, the patient may be treated with medication such as alpha-blockers to relax the bladder neck or 5-alpha reductase inhibitors to decrease the size of the prostate. The patient may be referred back to the therapist for treatment for his urge urinary incontinence. The therapist could then give the patient pelvic floor muscle exercises with biofeedback, teach urge-suppression techniques, and provide advice on fluid adjustment.

(4) A young man is sent to the GP by his partner to be treated for his severe urinary urgency.

Q. What could be the possible causes of his urinary urgency?

A. He may be suffering from urgency due to:
   (a) high caffeine intake
   (b) high alcoholic intake
   (c) urethritis
   (d) cystitis
   (e) idiopathic detrusor overactivity
   (f) detrusor overactivity due to a neurological condition

(5) A patient is sent to you with post-micturition dribble.

Q. What advice would you give him?

A. He should be taught to contract his pelvic floor muscles strongly after he has completed micturition to eject the urine from the bulbar portion of his urethra. He should also be taught pelvic floor muscle exercises in order to strengthen the bulbocavernosus muscle, which eliminates the last few drops of urine.

SUMMARY

Frequency, nocturia, urgency, urge urinary incontinence, stress urinary incontinence, post-micturition dribble and post-prostatectomy incontinence can be treated conservatively. Treatment modalities include pelvic floor muscle exercises, biofeedback, electrical treatment, lifestyle changes and urge suppression. Treatment progression is patient-specific and dependent on ongoing assessment.

10 Literature Review of Treatment before and after Prostatectomy

Key points

- A literature review revealed nine RCTs using pelvic floor muscle for post-prostatectomy incontinence.
- Grade II evidence showed that pelvic floor exercises seem to have merit as a treatment for post-prostatectomy incontinence.

INTRODUCTION

Transurethral resection of prostate may be performed for bladder outlet obstruction caused by benign prostatic hyperplasia, and radical prostatectomy may be performed for prostate cancer.

Complications following prostate surgery include urinary incontinence and erectile dysfunction. The internal urethral sphincter at the bladder neck is damaged in all forms of prostatectomy and continence relies on a competent external urethral sphincter, reinforced by pelvic floor musculature. Following transurethral resection of prostate and radical prostatectomy, patients may have iatrogenic stress incontinence due to sphincter damage, or urge incontinence, or a combination of both types. The Prostate Cancer Outcomes Study, using a sample of 1,291 men with localised prostate cancer living in six regions of the USA, showed that 18 months or more after radical prostatectomy 8.4 % of men still suffered from urinary incontinence and 59.9 % from erectile dysfunction (Stanford et al. 2000). The impotent men who were potent pre-surgery included 65 % of non-nerve-sparing procedures, 58 % of unilateral nerve-sparing and 56 % of bilateral nerve-sparing.

The pelvic floor muscles have a tripartite function: (i) they support the contents of the abdominal cavity; (ii) they control the bladder and bowel functions; and (iii) they have an important function during sexual activity. In normal men, the paired ischiocavernosus muscles increase the intracavernosal pressure in the tumescent penis to achieve full rigidity. The bulbocavernosus muscle has two functions: (i) it eliminates the last few drops of urine following micturition; and (ii) it expels the seminal fluid by rhythmic contractions resulting in ejaculation.

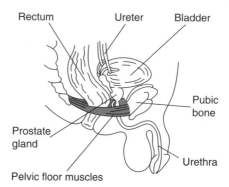

Figure 10.1. Male pelvic floor muscles (Reproduced by permission of NEEN Mobilis Healthcare Group. *Source*: Dorey, 2004b)

Treatment follows a full subjective and objective assessment which includes a digital anal examination in which the strength and endurance of the anal sphincter and the puborectalis muscle is recorded.

Men can be encouraged to tighten and lift the pelvic floor muscles as in the control of flatus or the prevention of urine flow and can practise in front of a mirror to observe a visible retraction of the base of the penis into the body and a testicular lift. The amount and progression of pelvic floor exercise is determined by individual assessment and digital anal examination.

A literature review was conducted to explore whether pelvic floor muscle exercises were a realistic first-line conservative approach for the treatment of post-prostatectomy urinary incontinence.

LITERATURE SEARCH

A literature search of randomised controlled trials (RCTs) was undertaken to ascertain whether pelvic floor muscle training had merit as a treatment to relieve incontinence in men after prostatectomy.

LITERATURE SEARCH STRATEGY

A search of the following computerised databases from 1980 to 2005 was undertaken: Medline, AAMED (Allied and Alternative Medicine), CINAHL, EMBASE – Rehabilitation and Physical Medicine, and The Cochrane Library Database. The keywords chosen were: *urinary incontinence; continence; post-prostatectomy incontinence; conservative treatment; physical therapy; physiotherapy; pelvic floor exercises; pelvic floor muscle training; Kegel exer-*

cises; biofeedback. A manual search was undertaken of identified manuscripts reporting on research studies gained from the references of this literature.

SELECTION CRITERIA

Only randomised controlled trials which reported the results of pelvic floor muscle training to restore pelvic floor function in men before or after prostatectomy were included provided they used reliable and relevant outcome measures.

METHODOLOGICAL QUALITY

Methodological rigour was assessed from the hierarchy of evidence used by the International Continence Society (Table 10.1).

RESULTS

The results from the literature review showed that the treatment of male urinary incontinence by physical therapists has been based on the evidence from a few randomised controlled trials using pelvic floor muscle training (Table 10.2).

One level II RCT was identified which used pelvic floor muscle exercises before and after TURP compared to a control group. At 3 weeks post TURP there were significantly fewer urinary incontinence episodes in the active group.

Four level II RCTs were identified which used pelvic floor muscle exercises to treat urinary incontinence before and after radical prostatectomy compared to a control group. Of these, two RCTs identified a significant difference to the continence outcomes between the groups post surgery.

Table 10.1. Levels of evidence (Adapted from Sackett 1986)

I	Strong evidence from at least one systematic review of multiple well-designed randomised controlled trials
II	Strong evidence from at least one properly designed randomised controlled trial of appropriate size
III	Evidence from well-designed trials such as non-randomised trials, cohort studies, time series or matched case-control studies
IV	Evidence from well-designed non-experimental studies from more than one centre or research group
V	Opinions of respected authorities, based on the clinical evidence, descriptive studies or reports of expert committees

Table 10.2. Review of RCTs using pelvic floor muscle training before and after prostatectomy

Author/design	Subjects	Method	Outcomes
Hunter et al. (2004) *The Cochrane Library* **Level I evidence**	8 RCTs post radical prostatectomy, 1 RCT post TURP and 1 RCT after both	PFMT Biofeedback Electrical stimulation Lifestyle adjustment	There may be some benefit in offering pelvic floor exercises in the early postoperative period **Subjective and objective outcomes**
Mathewson-Chapman (1997) *Journal of Cancer Education* **Level II evidence**	Randomised 26 men mean age 60 post radical prostatectomy to intervention group and 24 men mean age 60 to control group	Intervention group 1 pre-op PFMT and BFB PFMT and home BFB for 3 to 12 weeks after surgery Control group 1 pre-op PFMT and BFB only Outcome measures Questionnaire Number of pads 24-hour pad test	**Drop-outs 2/53 At 2, 5 and 12 weeks postoperatively** No differences between groups in number of pads **Subjective and objective outcomes**
Moore et al. (1999) *British Journal of Urology International*	18 men mean age 67.4 post radical prostatectomy randomised to intervention group 1, 19 men mean age 65.7 to	Intervention group 1 Post-op PFMT for 12 weeks Intervention 2 PFMT for 12 weeks + electrical stimulation	**Drop-outs 5/63 At 8, 12, 16 and 24 weeks post-op** No significant difference in incontinence between groups

			Subjective and objective outcomes
Level II evidence	intervention group 2, 21 men mean age 66.8 to control group	<u>Control group</u> Post-op written and verbal PFMT <u>Outcome measures</u> 24-hour pad test QoL questionnaire Number of leaks	
Bales et al. (2000) *Urology* **Level II evidence**	50 men mean age 59.3 randomised to pre-radical prostatectomy group and 50 men mean age 60.9 to control group	<u>Intervention group</u> 2 to 4 sessions pre-op PFMT and BFB + pre- and post-op home exercises <u>Control group</u> Post-op written and verbal PFMT <u>Outcome measures</u> Number of pads	**Drop-outs 3/100** **At 1, 2, 3, 4 or 6 months** No significant difference between groups **Objective outcomes**
Franke et al. (2000) *Journal of Urology* **Level II evidence**	15 men mean age 62.3 post radical prostatectomy randomised to intervention group and 15 men mean age 60.7 to control group	<u>Intervention group</u> 5 sessions PFMT + BFB <u>Control group</u> No treatment <u>Outcome measures</u> Voiding diary 48-hour pad test	**Drop-outs at 24 weeks 50%** **At 6 weeks, 3 and 6 months** No significant difference between groups **Objective outcomes**

Table 10.2. *Continued*

Author/design	Subjects	Method	Outcomes
Van Kampen et al. (2000) *Lancet* **Level II evidence**	50 men mean age 64.4 post radical prostatectomy randomised to intervention group and 52 men mean age 66.6 to control group	<u>Intervention group</u> PFMT + BFB <u>Control group</u> Placebo electrical stimulation <u>Outcome measures</u> 24-hour and 1-hour pad tests Voiding chart IPSS Number of pads	**Drop-outs 4/100** **At 1, 6 and 12 months post-op** Significant between group difference in duration ($p < 0.001$) and severity of incontinence ($p = 0.001$) **Subjective and objective outcomes**
Parekh et al. (2003) *Journal of Urology* **Level II evidence**	19 men post radical prostatectomy mean age 61.6 randomised to intervention group and 19 men mean age 55.5 to control group	<u>Intervention group</u> 2 sessions pre-op PFMT + BFB Post-op PFMT <u>Control group</u> No treatment <u>Outcome measures</u> Number of pads Questionnaire	**Drop-outs 2/38** **At 12 weeks** Intervention group improved significantly ($p < 0.05$) **At 6, 16, 20, 28 and 52 weeks** No significant difference between groups **Subjective and objective outcomes**
Joseph & Chang (2000) *Urologic Nursing*	1 man post TURP and 10 men post radical prostatectomy randomised to	<u>Intervention group</u> PFMT and BFB <u>Control group</u> Verbal teaching + digital	**At 4 weeks** No significant difference between groups

Level II evidence	intervention or control group	anal assessment Outcome measures 24-hour pad test Voiding diary and IIQ-7	Subjective and objective outcomes
Porru et al. (2001) *Neurourology and Urodynamics* **Level II evidence**	30 men pre TURP mean age 66 randomised to intervention group and 28 men mean age 66 to control group	Intervention group 1 pre-op PFMT session PFMT after catheter removal Control group Verbal and written PFMT Outcome measures AUA Symptom Score ICS*male* Voiding diaries QoL questionnaire	**Drop-outs 3/58** **At 3 weeks post catheter removal** Intervention group 4 incontinence episodes ($p < 0.01$) Post-micturition dribble ($p < 0.01$) Digital anal grade improved from 2.8 to 3.8 ($p < 0.01$) Control group 12 incontinence episodes **At 4 weeks post catheter removal** No significant difference **Subjective and objective outcomes**
Sueppel et al. (2001) *Urologic Nursing* **Level II evidence**	8 men mean age 61.8 post radical prostatectomy randomised to intervention group and 8 men mean age 61.1 to control group	Intervention group 2 sessions pre-op PFMT PFMT + BFB 6 weeks post-op Control group PFMT + BFB 6 weeks post-op Outcome measures 45-minute pad test at 1 year Questionnaire Voiding diary	**Drop-outs not mentioned** **At 1 year** Intervention group Significant improvement Mean pad weight 2.8 g Control group Mean pad weight 33.3 g **Subjective and objective outcomes**

Key: PFMT = pelvic floor muscle training; BFB = biofeedback; IIQ-7 = International Incontinence Questionnaire-7; AUA = American Urological Association; ICS = International Continence Society; QoL = quality of life.

Four level II RCTs were identified which compared pelvic floor exercises to a control group in the treatment of urinary incontinence after radical prostatectomy. Of these, only one RCT found a significant difference in continence outcomes between the groups.

No RCTs were found which specifically treated post-prostatectomy urge urinary incontinence.

EVIDENCE FOR THE EFFECT

One Cochrane Review of 10 randomised controlled trials was found which used conservative treatment in the treatment of men following radical prostatectomy and provided level I evidence (Hunter et al. 2004). The five RCTs using pelvic floor muscle training as the principal intervention in this review were identified in the literature search and are discussed below individually.

The literature search revealed nine randomised controlled trials each providing level II evidence using pelvic floor muscle training in the treatment of men with urinary incontinence (Table 10.2). Of these, one trial explored pelvic floor muscle training before and after TURP (Porru et al. 2001). Four trials explored pelvic floor muscle training before and after radical prostatectomy (Bales et al. 2000; Mathewson-Chapman, 1997; Parekh et al. 2003; Sueppel et al. 2001). Four trials explored pelvic floor muscle training post radical prostatectomy (Franke et al. 2000; Joseph & Chang 2000; Moore et al. 1999; Van Kampen et al. 2000).

EFFECT SIZE

Four trials demonstrated a significant difference in the reduction of incontinence between the PFMT group and the control group (Parekh et al. 2003; Porru et al. 2001; Sueppel et al. 2001; Van Kampen et al. 2000).

CLINICAL SIGNIFICANCE

Two RCTs used pad tests to demonstrate a clinically significant reduction in the amount of urinary leakage (Sueppel et al. 2001; Van Kampen et al. 2000).

METHODOLOGICAL QUALITY

The trials for men with post-prostatectomy urinary incontinence, which failed to demonstrate an improvement, were of varying methodological quality. The majority of trials used small sample sizes. Unfortunately, five trials gave the control group a list of pelvic floor muscle exercises which compromised the treatment effect (Bales et al. 2000; Joseph & Chang 2000; Mathewson-

Chapman 1997; Moore et al. 1999; Porru et al. 2001). One trial recruited men a mean of 18.9 weeks (range: 4 to 241 weeks) after radical prostatectomy with four subjects recruited more than two years after surgery who were randomised to one of the intervention groups (Moore et al. 1999). Pelvic floor muscle training should be commenced before surgery and aimed at an early return to continence.

Outcome measures varied between the trials. Only one trial used digital anal grades to record pelvic floor muscle strength (Porru et al. 2001). Most studies failed to assess pelvic floor muscle strength prior to surgery. The days to continence were not always measured by validated outcome measures, pad tests, voiding diaries or validated quality of life questionnaires. The severity of incontinence was objectively assessed by a 45-minute, 1-hour, or 24-hour pad test in three trials (Moore et al. 1999; Sueppel et al. 2001; Van Kampen et al. 2000).

Most trials recorded the drop-out rate, which was low in most cases; but one trial had a drop-out rate at 24 weeks of 50%, which must have compromised the results (Franke et al. 2000).

TYPE OF INTERVENTION

The treatment protocol varied and, in most trials, failed to include guarding the pelvic floor muscles during activities which increased intra-abdominal pressure. Men were encouraged to use their pelvic floor muscles during activity such as coughing, sneezing, rising from sitting, laughing, shouting and lifting in one successful trial (Van Kampen et al. 2000). It was not stated in most trials whether maximal pelvic floor muscle contractions were taught to gain muscle strength and hypertrophy plus some less-intensive, sustained contractions for endurance.

Most trials used biofeedback to enhance the effect of pelvic floor exercises, although this possible additional effect was inconclusive (Bales et al. 2000; Franke et al. 2000; Joseph & Chang 2000; Mathewson-Chapman 1997; Parekh et al. 2003; Sueppel et al. 2001; Van Kampen et al. 2000). In one trial, one pre-operative session of biofeedback failed to make a difference especially as both groups were practising home exercises before and after radical prostatectomy (Bales et al. 2000).

No trials recorded treatment of urge incontinence using urge-suppression techniques.

FREQUENCY AND DURATION OF TRAINING

The length of treatment ranged from 3 to 12 weeks, although all trials stressed the importance of regular home exercises. The exercise regime varied and there is a need for a standardised pelvic floor muscle training programme. The training programme is dependent on the quality of the physiotherapist and the assessment of specific patient needs. Patient education is paramount so that the patient becomes a willing partner in the delivery of healthcare and adheres to the advice given. Specific advice may be given concerning exercise positions, number of repetitions, strength of the contractions, and pelvic floor muscle work during activities. Other advice concerns fluid intake, weight reduction, smoking cessation and urge-suppression techniques.

The duration of training was only minimal prior to prostatectomy, and in some trials absent. There is difficulty providing the required amount of pre-operative pelvic floor muscle training for men who undergo immediate surgery for cancer. However, even one session of pelvic floor muscle training has been shown to be better than none (Porru et al. 2001). As the bladder neck sphincter is damaged in all forms of prostatectomy, continence relies on an effective external urinary sphincter enhanced by the surrounding pelvic floor muscles. If these muscles are weak and not used effectively during the period of prostatic blockage, urinary leakage is more likely to occur when the blockage is removed.

SHORT- AND LONG-TERM EFFECTS

Outcome measures were recorded from 1 week after surgery to 12 months. Urinary incontinence was significantly improved at 1, 2 and 3 weeks (Porru et al. 2001), 1 month (Van Kampen et al. 2000), 3 months (Parekh et al. 2003), 6 months (Van Kampen et al. 2000), and one year (Sueppel et al. 2001; Van Kampen et al. 2000). Weak pelvic floor muscles may take 3 to 6 months to strengthen to full fitness. Also, pelvic floor muscle action helps tissue viability and healing by increasing the local blood supply.

PSYCHOSEXUAL ISSUES

Psychosexual issues were not addressed in any of these trials.

ADVERSE EFFECTS

In one trial, one subject experienced rectal pain whilst performing pelvic floor exercises and discontinued treatment (Moore et al. 1999). Rectal pain should be treated before pelvic floor exercises are resumed as these exercises should not be uncomfortable.

RECOMMENDATIONS BASED ON EVIDENCE

There is level II evidence that pelvic floor muscle exercises are effective for an early return to continence after both TURP and radical prostatectomy. Pelvic floor muscle training should include some maximal work for increasing and maintaining strength, some less intensive work to increase muscle endurance and, importantly, regular functional work during activities which increase intra-abdominal pressure.

PREVENTION OF URINARY INCONTINENCE

There were no randomised controlled trials exploring whether pelvic floor muscle training can prevent urinary incontinence. It is reasonable to suppose that if pelvic floor muscle training relieves urinary incontinence then strengthening these muscles prior to surgery may well prevent urinary leakage. It may also help to prevent erectile dysfunction (Chapter 15). However, to be effective pelvic floor muscles should be used regularly during functional activities.

CONCLUSIONS

There is grade II level evidence that pelvic floor muscle exercises seem to have merit as a treatment for post-prostatectomy incontinence. Four trials out of nine randomised controlled trials demonstrated a significant difference in the reduction of incontinence between the group receiving pelvic floor muscle training and the control group. This level II evidence showed that early return to urinary continence was found in some men who performed pelvic floor exercises before and after TURP and before and after radical prostatectomy.

The trials for men with post-prostatectomy urinary incontinence, which found no difference between the groups, were of varying methodological quality. Trials used small sample sizes and some trials gave the control group a list of pelvic floor exercises, which compromised the treatment effect.

There was no evidence that biofeedback enhanced the treatment effect.

The duration of training was only minimal prior to prostatectomy, and in some trials absent. The treatment protocol varied and in some trials failed to include guarding the pelvic floor muscles during activities which increased intra-abdominal pressure. The days to continence were not always measured by validated outcome measures, pad tests, urinary diaries or validated quality of life questionnaires.

For those patients who appear to have been cured or improved with pelvic floor muscle training, it may be prudent to continue these simple exercises for life and possibly avoid a return of incontinence. The same exercises may also help men suffering from erectile dysfunction. To gain long-term compliance, it may be possible to maintain muscle performance with a minimal exercise programme.

A multi-centred randomised controlled trial with larger sample numbers is needed to explore the use of pelvic floor exercises before and after all forms of prostatectomy.

11 Treatment of Post-prostatectomy Patients

Key points

- Following prostatectomy many men have stress incontinence and some men have urge incontinence.
- Stress urinary incontinence may be treated with pelvic floor muscle exercises and include tightening the pelvic floor muscles during times of increased intra-abdominal pressure.
- Frequency, nocturia, urgency and urge urinary incontinence can be treated with pelvic floor muscle exercises, urge-suppression techniques and lifestyle changes.
- Pelvic floor muscle exercises should be the first line treatment for men with erectile dysfunction.

INTRODUCTION

Post-prostatectomy incontinence should be treated according to the presenting symptoms. Following TURP and radical prostatectomy, patients may have stress urinary incontinence due to sphincter damage, or urge urinary incontinence, or a combination of both types. They may also have post-micturition dribble – but they may well have experienced this before surgery.

The internal urethral sphincter at the bladder neck is damaged in all forms of prostatectomy and continence relies on a competent external urethral sphincter, reinforced by the pelvic floor musculature. The external urethral sphincter may be weakened from disuse during the period when the urethra was compressed by an enlarged prostate.

Symptoms of frequency, nocturia, urgency, urge urinary incontinence, stress urinary incontinence and post-micturition dribble can be treated conservatively. Treatment modalities include pelvic floor muscle exercises, biofeedback, urge-suppression techniques, electrical treatment and lifestyle changes.

ASSESSMENT

Treatment follows a full subjective assessment, which includes a full surgical and medical history (see the Appendix). For patients who have had a radical prostatectomy, it is important to know whether the patient has undergone nerve-sparing surgery. The objective assessment includes a digital anal examination in which the strength and endurance and speed of recruitment of the anal sphincter and the puborectalis muscle is assessed and recorded. These muscles are graded 0–6 for muscle strength using a modified Oxford scale, for the duration of the hold in seconds and for the ability to perform a fast contraction (Chapter 8).

PATIENT EDUCATION

Most men appreciate an explanation of their medical condition with the help of diagrams and models and the treatment options available.

TREATMENT

PRE-OPERATIVE TREATMENT

Two studies have reinforced the use of pre-prostatectomy pelvic floor muscle exercises at a time when patients are fit and able to cope with learning a new skill (Sueppel et al. 2001; Porru et al. 2001). Also there is likely to be a positive benefit from an early established patient/therapist relationship.

PELVIC FLOOR MUSCLE EXERCISES

Men should practise pelvic floor muscle exercises as soon as they know that they may need prostate surgery. After surgery pelvic floor exercises may be performed gently immediately after surgery while the catheter is in place provided the surgeon agrees. When the catheter has been removed pelvic floor muscle exercises may be performed more strongly. Pelvic floor exercises should be individually taught to make sure the patient is lifting up the pelvic floor and not bearing down as if defaecating (i.e. performing a valsalva manoeuvre). Men can be encouraged to tighten and lift the pelvic floor muscles as in the control of flatus and the prevention of urine flow and can practise in front of a mirror to observe a visible retraction of the base of the penis into the body and a testicular lift. The testicular lift may be sluggish initially. In some men with weak pelvic floor muscles only one testicle might rise initially. As the pelvic floor muscles strengthen both testicles will lift more quickly to a higher level. Also, patients can be taught to palpate a contraction of the ischiocavernosus muscle at the perineum 2 cm medially and 2 cm anteriorly to the ischial tuberosity.

The convenient positions for practising pelvic floor muscle exercises are supine lying with knees bent and the knees apart; standing with feet apart;

and sitting with knees apart. The intensity of the contraction is more important than the frequency as maximum voluntary effort causes muscle hypertrophy and increased muscle strength (Dinubile 1991; Guyton 1986). In order to achieve full fitness, pelvic floor muscle training should include exercises for endurance as well as for muscle strength by submaximal contractions (Guyton 1986). Muscle training, therefore, depends on the motivation of the patient and the adherence to the pelvic floor exercise regimen (Jackson et al. 1996). Treatment progression is patient-specific and dependent on ongoing assessment.

There has been no research conducted to give a clear indication of the number of pelvic floor muscle exercises needed to build up muscle bulk, strength and endurance. Kegel (1956) instructed female patients to perform about 300 contractions a day. For muscle building, it is the quality not the quantity that is important. Home exercises can be practised as strongly as possible twice a day in supine lying, sitting and standing. The hold time in seconds is set individually by the therapist according to the number of seconds held during the digital anal examination. The rest time should exceed the hold time to allow the muscle to recover from exertion. Randomised controlled trials are needed to ascertain the number of repetitions needed to gain optimum relief of symptoms.

PELVIC FLOOR MUSCLE EXERCISES FOR STRESS URINARY INCONTINENCE

After prostatectomy, men frequently report that they do not leak urine during sitting, and lying but only on changing position especially rising from sitting and bending forwards. Both these activities increase intra-abdominal pressure. Men can be taught to rise from sitting without bending forwards and whilst tightening their pelvic floor muscles. 'The knack' of tightening at times of increased intra-abdominal pressure should be taught to cope with activities such as moving from sitting to standing, coughing, sneezing and lifting (Miller et al. 1996). Training is moving towards more functional exercises with emphasis on the voluntary use of the muscles during times when they would normally contract by reflex activity. Regular voluntary use during certain activities may well become an automatic action.

Men can be taught to lift their pelvic floor slightly whilst walking. Instruction to tighten the anal sphincter about 50 % of maximum whilst walking will achieve this supportive lift which can become part of good posture and way of carrying oneself.

Manometric (pressure) or EMG biofeedback is a useful adjunct to pelvic floor muscle re-education to stimulate greater patient effort.

Electrical stimulation may assist in showing patients how to initially contract the pelvic floor muscles for men with a grade 0–1 muscle contraction who have had a TURP. Electrical stimulation is contraindicated in patients who have or have had prostate cancer as we do not know if electrical stimulation will cause a proliferation of abnormal cells. The contraindications for electrical stimulation are shown in Chapter 9.

PELVIC FLOOR MUSCLE EXERCISES FOR URGE URINARY INCONTINENCE

Pelvic floor muscle exercises can be used for urge urinary incontinence to strengthen the pelvic floor musculature and regain the ability to control the urge to void urine. It is suggested that when the pelvic floor contracts the detrusor muscle relaxes due to the activity of the perineopudendal facilitative reflex (Mahony et al. 1977). It is believed that pelvic floor muscle training leads to increased muscle tone which guards against unwanted detrusor contractions, although there are no trials to support this theory.

Lower urinary tract symptoms, especially frequency, urgency, urge incontinence and nocturia, are significantly associated with sexual dysfunction in men (Frankel et al. 1998). The filling symptoms of frequency, nocturia, urgency and urge urinary incontinence can be treated with pelvic floor muscle exercises, urge-suppression techniques and lifestyle changes, including avoiding constipation and fluid intake advice.

Severe urge incontinence may be treated with anticholinergic medication. The unwanted side-effects of this medication that may occur include a dry mouth, drowsiness, blurred vision and constipation.

Men should be advised to drink about 1½ litres (3 pints) a day. More fluid is necessary when exercising, after eating salty foods and in a hot climate. Water is the best thirst-quencher. Alcohol and caffeine can make the bladder more irritable. Headaches and other unpleasant symptoms may occur if the caffeine is not reduced gradually over a 3-week period.

Smoking increases detrusor overactivity and is linked to urge incontinence (Haidinger et al. 2000). Smokers may be helped to quit by joining a smoking cessation programme, run at most GP practices, or by telephoning in the UK the NHS smoking helpline: 0800 169 0169.

PELVIC FLOOR MUSCLE EXERCISES FOR POST-MICTURITION DRIBBLE

Post-micturition dribble is not solely a condition of post-prostatectomy patients but a common condition amongst men of all ages (see Chapter 6). It is common for men to experience leakage of a few drops of urine after urination when walking away from the toilet. It has been shown in recent research that tightening the pelvic floor muscles up strongly after the completion of voiding whilst standing poised over the toilet expels the last few drops from the bulbar U-shaped portion of the urethra and eliminates post-micturition dribble (Dorey et al. 2004b). This strong post-void pelvic floor muscle contraction supersedes the technique of milking the urine from the bulbar urethra with bulbar urethral massage.

OUTCOMES

Pelvic floor muscle exercises aim to achieve urinary control, continence and confidence in conjunction with other conservative measures. However, it is not always possible to gain this outcome and patients may need help managing their condition. It is important to set realistic goals.

POST-PROSTATECTOMY COMPLICATIONS

Various postoperative complications may arise after prostatectomy (Table 11.1) and can be treated by different members of the healthcare team. The most serious complications are a high temperature indicative of infection and retention of urine which can lead to overstretching the detrusor muscle and the possibility of kidney damage.

INCONTINENCE PADS

Incontinence pads held in place with tight-fitting pants are preferable to a penile sheath and leg bag urine collection system. Men should be encouraged to attempt to pass urine regularly and not rely on a pad or drainage system. It is important to encourage the bladder storage phase of micturition. Men should be encouraged to tighten their pelvic floor muscles when they have a sensation of leakage of urine or at times when leakage may occur to try and control the leakage.

Table 11.1. Problems which may arise following prostatectomy

Problem post-surgery	Professional help
Bleeding from incision wound	GP or practice nurse
Wound infection	GP or practice nurse
High temperature	See GP immediately
Blood in the urine	GP or practice nurse
Retention of urine	See urologist or GP immediately
Pain in the pelvic area	GP or practice nurse
Pain during urination	GP or practice nurse
Incontinence of urine	Specialist continence physiotherapist Continence nurse specialist
Problem with pad absorbency	Continence advisor
Erectile dysfunction	Visit erectile dysfunction clinic Specialist continence physiotherapist

PERSISTING INCONTINENCE

Patients with long-term post-prostatectomy incontinence may still benefit by using pelvic floor muscle exercises a year after surgery. One man who commenced pelvic floor exercises a year after radical prostatectomy kept a chart of his monthly urinary leakage (Figure 11.1). He is still continuing to improve and gains encouragement from the continued patient/therapist relationship. He regretted not reading the booklet 'Living and Loving after Prostate Surgery' prior to his radical prostatectomy and not knowing about pelvic floor muscle exercises at that stage (Dorey 2005).

There are a number of surgical options to help men with severe incontinence which persists for more than a year after radical prostatectomy. There is a new Proact device, which can be implanted under minimally invasive surgery, or male sling surgery for men with persisting incontinence. These are alternatives to the more major artificial urethral sphincter.

RETROGRADE EJACULATION

After TURP, some men experience retrograde ejaculation, when the semen enters the bladder at ejaculation. This is due to the loss of the bladder neck sphincter and the semen is passed with the next urination.

URETHRAL STRICTURE

After a radical prostatectomy, a urethral stricture may form during the healing process at the anastomosis between the bladder and the urethra. This stric-

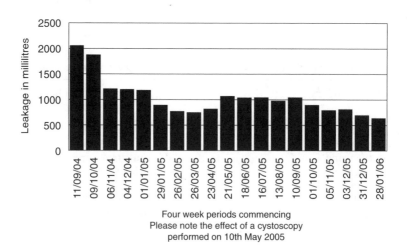

Figure 11.1. Monthly urinary leakage during pelvic floor muscle training commenced one year after prostatectomy

ture may cause obstruction to the flow of urine. Treatment consists of stretching the urethra under anaesthetic or surgical resection. Maintenance treatment consists of passing a lubricated catheter along the urethra at regular intervals. Occasionally a urethral stricture may prevent the urethra from closing during a contraction of the external urethral sphincter.

POST-PROSTATECTOMY ERECTILE DYSFUNCTION

Some men who were sexually active before their prostatectomy will be able to resume a normal sex life. However, some men may find that they have difficulties gaining or maintaining an erection. This may be due to surgical nerve involvement or postoperative swelling leading to nerve compression. Damaged nerves can regrow and healing continues for up to a year after prostatectomy. Healing takes place better if there is a good blood supply. Pelvic floor muscle exercises help to bring more oxygenated blood to the area and help to remove de-oxygenated blood. Also, general exercise such as walking up hills or stairs or playing sports such as golf helps to improve cardiovascular fitness.

Pelvic floor exercises may help to improve erectile function. One of the first signs that erectile function is improving is when men wake up with an erection. Pelvic floor exercises need to be practised daily for up to 6 months for men with erectile dysfunction, though it is prudent for all men to practise a few strong contractions every day.

Pelvic floor muscle exercises designed to improve incontinence may also help to alleviate erectile dysfunction. There are no trials which have monitored the effect of pelvic floor exercises on the erectile function of men after prostatectomy. In some centres men following radical prostatectomy are treated with oral medication to achieve an erection to kick-start the normal erectile mechanism. Other treatment options for post-prostatectomy patients with erectile dysfunction include topical therapies (penile creams containing medicated drugs), vacuum devices, constriction bands, intra-urethral drugs, intracavernous injections, and more rarely penile vein surgery and penile implants. Couples may be referred to an erectile dysfunction clinic to discuss the use of any of these treatment options in order to choose the best option for their needs (Chapter 15).

Some men leak urine at orgasm. Men are advised to empty their bladder before sexual activity.

A LOVING RELATIONSHIP

Men and women have different sexual needs. A loving relationship may take the form of sharing, closeness, touching and cuddling. Some couples are content without sexual intercourse. Those in close relationships respect the wishes and needs of their partners. Partners may wish to satisfy each other. Sexual activity does not have to include sexual intercourse as couples may prefer mutual fondling, stroking, manual and oral stimulation.

Help is available at sexual dysfunction clinics for those men who feel devastated, depressed or just saddened by their lack of erections. Couples are encouraged to attend together so that they can choose the best method that is appropriate for them. Problems of incontinence and erectile difficulties can be shared, and discussed jointly; advice can be sought and treatment commenced to help improve the quality of life for both partners. This may be the beginning of a new, shared stage of living and loving.

SUMMARY

Post-prostatectomy stress urinary incontinence may be treated with pelvic floor muscle exercises and should include tightening the pelvic floor muscles during times of increased intra-abdominal pressure. The filling symptoms of frequency, nocturia, urgency and urge urinary incontinence can be treated with pelvic floor muscle exercises, urge-suppression techniques and lifestyle changes, including advice on avoiding constipation and fluid intake advice. Pelvic floor muscle exercises should be the first-line treatment for men with erectile dysfunction.

FREQUENTLY ASKED QUESTIONS

What is stress urinary incontinence?

Stress urinary incontinence is leakage of urine which occurs on exertion, when there is an increase in pressure inside your abdomen. It may happen after prostate surgery when you are rising from sitting, bending, coughing, sneezing, shouting, laughing or lifting.

If I tighten my pelvic floor muscles during activities which increase internal abdominal pressure, will this become automatic?

Strengthening the pelvic floor muscles will lead to increased resting tone in the muscles which support the pelvic floor. If you tighten before and during every time you perform activities which increase your internal abdominal pressure, it will become an automatic reaction.

I have a severe uncontrollable urge to visit the toilet, is there some medication which can help?

There is anticholinergic medication for men with severe, uncontrollable urges to pass urine. Your GP will prescribe this. Strengthening the pelvic floor muscles and practising urge-suppression techniques also helps to reduce this problem. It may help you to gradually reduce your caffeine intake over a 3-week period and quit smoking.

How do I know my pelvic floor muscles are stronger?

Your specialist continence physiotherapist can perform a gentle digital anal examination to let you know your pelvic floor muscle grade. Other markers are a reduction in the amount or frequency of urinary leakage.

Can I use Viagra to kick-start my erections?

Viagra is sometimes prescribed after prostate surgery for men who are unable to gain an erection. This may well kick-start natural erections. Pelvic floor exercises can help to restore the ability to regain and maintain normal erections. Waking with an erection in the morning is a good sign that your erections are returning.

12 Medication

Key points

- Medication may be used in conjunction with physical therapy for a number of urological conditions such as detrusor overactivity, nocturnal enuresis, nocturia and benign prostatic hyperplasia.
- Some medication has an adverse effect on lower urinary tract function.

INTRODUCTION

It is estimated that in England there were around 21,700 nurses able to prescribe from the Nurse Prescribing Formulary, and around 2,400 qualified to prescribe from the Extended Nurse Prescribing Formulary and supplementary prescribing. District Nurses and Health Visitors (Independent Nurse Prescribers) who have completed the necessary training can only prescribe the preparations listed in Part XVIIB(i) of the Drug Tariff. The list includes almost all appliances (including wound management products) and reagents listed in Part IX.

Extended and Supplementary Nurse Prescribers can also prescribe from the list of products in Part XVIIB(ii) of the Drug Tariff. This list includes all licensed Pharmacy and General Sale List medicines prescribable on the NHS for a specified list of medical conditions together with a list of Prescription Only Medicines (POM). The list of POMs includes some controlled drugs such as codeine phosphate and dihydrocodeine tartrate. Supplementary prescribers can prescribe all General Sales List medicines, all POMs (except controlled drugs), medicines for use outside their licence indications and unlicensed drugs provided they are included within a patient-specific clinical management plan.

In April 2005, the statutory instrument laid before Parliament gave supplementary prescribing rights to physiotherapists, which applies to England, Wales, Scotland and Northern Ireland. Information is available on an information paper entitled 'Prescribing Rights for Physiotherapists' (Chartered Society of Physiotherapy, 2005).

Medication may be used in conjunction with physical therapy for a number of urological conditions such as detrusor overactivity, nocturnal enuresis, nocturia and benign prostatic hyperplasia.

PHARMACOTHERAPY FOR DETRUSOR OVERACTIVITY

Pharmacotherapy can be used in the management of detrusor overactivity to reduce involuntary detrusor contractions and increase functional bladder capacity. Antimuscarinics, also known as anticholinergics, are the most widely used treatment for overactive bladder and urinary urge incontinence (Andersson & Wein 2005). They may be useful for both moderate to severe urgency and moderate to severe urge urinary incontinence. This medication should always be used in conjunction with urge-suppression techniques and pelvic floor muscle exercises.

The main contraction of the bladder results from the release of acetylcholine and its action on muscarinic receptors. Muscarinic receptors are thought to be the primary mediators of human detrusor muscle contraction. To date five subtypes of muscarinic receptors have been identified using gene cloning techniques (M1–M5). Like most other smooth muscle, the bladder contains a mixed population of M2 and M3 muscarinic receptors; M2 constitute approximately 80 % and M3 account for 20 % of the total muscarinic receptor population but 100 % of the contractile response. There is some evidence that B3 adrenergic and M2 receptors may also have a role in active relaxation of the detrusor.

Antimuscarinic drugs are tertiary amines which block the muscarinic receptors within the detrusor muscle that mediate detrusor contraction in normal men. Bladder contractility is decreased and the bladder sphincter smooth muscle tone increased. However, drug therapy reduces detrusor overactivity but does not usually eliminate it (McGuire & O'Connell 1995). Voluntary and involuntary contractions are mediated mainly by acetylcholine-induced stimulation of muscarinic receptors. Antimuscarinic drugs will therefore depress both types of the contraction, irrespective of how the efferent part of the micturition reflex is activated (Keane & O'Sullivan 2000). Antimuscarinic drugs will also lower intravesical pressure, increase capacity and reduce the frequency of bladder contraction. They block the parasympathetic nerves, which control bladder voiding (Andersson & Wein 2005).

Data suggest that antimuscarinic drugs are well absorbed from the gastrointestinal tract and pass into the central nervous system (Dolman 2003). One of the main drawbacks to these agents is the side-effect profile: dry mouth due to the inhibition of salivary secretion, blurring of near vision (cycloplegia), tachycardia and inhibition of gut motility leading to constipation (Wein 1997). Urinary retention may be a further unwanted side-effect. One way to avoid many of the side-effects is to administer the drug intravesically, although this is often impracticable. All antimuscarinic drugs are contraindicated in narrow-angle glaucoma.

ANTIMUSCARINICS WITH BLADDER SPECIFICITY

Oxybutynin (Ditropan, Cystrin) is the most common prescribed treatment in the UK for overactive bladder. It is both antimuscarinic and a direct muscle relaxant. Its chief metobite, *N*-desethyl oxybutinin is also pharmacologically active and occurs in higher concentration than the parent compound. This metobite is thought to be responsible for the main adverse effects of this drug. As a tertiary amine it is well absorbed but undergoes an extensive first pass metabolism. Oxybutynin is also available in an extended release form (Lyrinel XL).

Oxybutynin transdermal patch (Kentera) the first and only transdermal treatment, it is a twice-weekly dosing schedule. The patch releases a dose of 3.9 mg of oxybutynin in 24 hours, bypassing the presystemetic gut wall metabolism with potential increased therapeutic levels with reduced side-effects.

Tolterodine (Detrusitol, Detrusitol XL) is a non-selective antimuscarinic, competitive antagonist with some functional selectivity for the bladder. This may explain why there is a lower incidence of dry mouth and a reduction in withdraws rate.

Propiverine (Detrunorm) has combined antimuscarinic and calcium channel blocking activity. 20 % of patients on propiverine report adverse side-effects, which are mainly anticholinergic in nature. Propiverine is rapidly absorbed but has a high first pass metabolism.

Trospium (Regurin) is an antimuscarinic derived from atropine (quaternary ammonium compound). It has no selectivity for muscarinic receptor subtypes and has a very low bioavailability of 5 %. It can achieve therapeutic levels within a week and has been shown to cause reduced cognitive problems compared to other antimuscarinics.

Solifenacin (Vesicare) is the latest to come onto the UK market. It is a long-acting muscarinic receptor antagonist developed for the treatment of detrusor overactivity.

Darafenacin (Emselex) is soon to be available in the UK and has gone through phase III studies here. It is a selective muscarinic M3 receptor and has no detectable effects on cognitive or cardiovascular function.

OTHER AGENTS

Imipramine (Tofrinil) is a tricyclic antidepressant which has anticholinergic, alpha-antagonistic, antihistamine, anti-5-HT and possible antidiuretic properties. It may be used in conjunction with oxybutynin in low doses. It is not licensed for use for an overactive bladder in the UK. It may help nocturnal enuresis. The side-effects of dry mouth, reflux oesophagitis, dry skin and visual accommodation difficulties are milder than those from oxybutynin.

However, the elderly may experience postural instability and drowsiness. It has the potential to cause cardiac arrhythmias. It may help co-existing stress incontinence due to its alpha-adrenergic profile but it is not licensed for this use in the UK.

Chilli derivatives such as capsaicin and resinferatoxin are undergoing investigation in their role in the treatment of detrusor overactivity. Published research on the outcomes of bladder instillation with capsaicin by De Ridder et al. (1997) showed that repeated instillation was effective in the treatment of detrusor overactivity. A single treatment was shown to last 3–6 months with 80 % of patients reporting a benefit. It does not have a recognised licence for bladder instillation.

Botox injected into the detrusor muscle is still in early stages for treating detrusor overactivity. The toxin acts by inhibiting acetylcholine release at the presynaptic cholinergic junction. Inhibiting acetylcholine release results in regionally decreased muscle contractility and muscle atrophy at the site of the injection. The chemical enervation that results is a reversible process as the axons resprout in approximately 3–6 months. Intravesical instillations of botulinum toxin A into the detrusor muscle is a promising treatment for detrusor overactivity when standard pharmacology has failed.

The Cochran report suggested that it is not yet clear whether bladder training is either more effective than drug treatment alone or useful as a supplement to drug treatment (Roe et al. 2002). Burgio (2002) suggested that combining approaches of behaviour and medication may result in better outcomes. All the options need to be considered and discussed with patients to find the most appropriate treatment for them. Antimuscarinic treatment does have a side-effect profile and it is for this reason that many patients discontinue treatment.

PHARMACOTHERAPY FOR STRESS URINARY INCONTINENCE

Duloxetine (Yentreve) is a selective serotonin and noradrenaline re-uptake inhibitor (SNRI) which works by improving external urinary sphincter tone and urethral closure pressure, and reducing urinary leakage. In preclinical studies, increased levels of 5-HT and NA in the sacral spinal cord lead to increased urethral contraction via enhanced pudendal nerve stimulation to the urethral striated sphincter muscle. The acetylcholine released by the pudendal nerve can then stimulate the receptors in the urethral sphincter to increase urethral sphincter contractility during the storage phase of the micturition cycle. Use with caution in patients with a history of mania, bipolar disorder or seizures, patients with increased intra-ocular pressure, or those at risk of acute narrow-angle glaucoma, patients taking anticoagulants or products known to affect platelet function and those with the tendency to bleed. The current licence is for the treatment of women with stress urinary incontinence, but trials are planned for post-prostatectomy patients with stress urinary incontinence.

PHARMACOTHERAPY FOR NOCTURNAL ENURESIS

First-line treatment is always correction of any underlying conditions, review of general health and current medication regime. In patients with peripheral oedema and/or congestive cardiac failure, fluid can pool in the lower limbs in the daytime and returns to the circulation at night. Appropriate management can prevent excessive variation in nocturnal intravesicular volume. There are limited studies on the effectiveness of such strategies as:

- fluid restriction in evening
- compression bandages
- restriction of caffeine and alcohol
- late-afternoon elevation of legs

MEDICATION FOR NOCTURIA

Diuretic treatment encouraging urine excretion before bedtime can be an option for nocturnal polyuria. Reynard et al. (1998) in a double-blind placebo-controlled trial, used Frusemide 6 hours before bedtime to reduce nocturia. Nocturnal voiding frequency and urine production were significantly reduced. *Desmopressin* may be used for nocturnal polyuria. Nocturnal polyuria may be due to loss of renal concentrating ability and the decreased production of antidiuretic hormone. Desmopressin (DDAVP) is a synthetic analogue of vasopressin and increases urine concentration and reduces total urine output. Side-effects of DDAVP should be balanced with the benefits as it can cause hyponatremia, oedema and heart failure (BNF), and is not licensed for the over-65 age group. Serum sodium levels should be checked 3 days after starting treatment or changing the dose.

Imipramine has been shown to decrease urine output in young adults. The effects of imipramine are thought to come from its alpha-adrenergic action on the proximal renal tubules with increased urea and water reabsorption (Hunsballe et al. 1997). Further work is needed to explore whether it has a similar effect on older adults.

Antiprostaglandin therapy may be prescribed using aspirin to reduce nocturia. Aspirin is a non-steroidal, anti-inflammatory drug (NSAID) with mild to moderate analgesic properties. Aspirin is also recognised as an anti-coagulant and antiprostaglandin as it blocks prostaglandin synthesis.

Treatment of nocturia requires accurate assessment of symptoms. Medication has a role once the cause of nocturia has been determined.

MEDICATION WHICH MAY HAVE AN ADVERSE EFFECT ON LOWER URINARY TRACT FUNCTION

Medication which may have an adverse effect on lower urinary tract function is listed in Table 12.1.

Table 12.1. Medication which may have an adverse effect on lower urinary tract function

Drug	Use	Effect
Alcohol	Social	Impairs mobility, reduces sensation, increases urinary frequency and urgency, induces diuresis
Anticholinesterase Neostigmine	Myasthenia gravis Irritable bowel spasm	Bladder sphincter muscle relaxation causing involuntary micturition Control of smooth muscle, increased peristalsis
Antimuscarinic drugs, also known as anticholinergics Benhexol Procyclidine Hyoscine Propantheline	Parkinson's disease Drug-induced Parkinsonism	Voiding difficulties
Drugs with antimuscarinic side-effects Antihistamines Pizotifen Promethazine	Allergies, hay fever, rashes, migraine, travel sickness	Voiding difficulties Reduced awareness of desire to void
Antidepressants Amitriptyline Lofepramide Imipramine	Depression	Voiding difficulties
Calcium channel blockers Nifedapine	Angina, arrhythmia, hypertension	Nocturia, increased frequency
Cytotoxics Cyclophosphamide Ifosfamide	Malignancies	Haemorrhagic cystitis

Table 12.1. *Continued*

Drug	Use	Effect
Diuretics		
Loop diuretics	Management of	
Frusemide	hypertension	Urinary urgency
Bumetanide	Pulmonary oedema	Urge urinary incontinence
Metazolone	Heart failure, oedema	
Thiazides	Diabetes insipidus	Urinary urgency
Bendrofluazide		Frequency
Cyclopenthiazide	Oliguria due to renal	
Amiloride,	failure	Urge urinary incontinence
Triamterene	Ascites, nephrotic	
Spironolactone	syndrome	
Hypnotics/sedatives		
Antipsychotics	Schizophrenia and	
Chlorpromazine	related psychotic	
Thioridazine	illness	Voiding difficulties, decreased
Droperidol,	Nausea, vomiting,	awareness
Haloperidol	agitation	
Pimozide	Anxiety	
Benzodiazepines		
Nitrazepam,	Sedation	Decreased awareness, impaired
Temazepam		mobility
Lorazepam		
Barbiturates		
Amylobarbitone	Sedation	Decreased awareness, impaired
Phenobarbitone		mobility
Chloral derivatives	Sedation	Decreased awareness, impaired
		mobility
Phenothiazines		
Chlorpromazine	Sedation	Decreased awareness of desire
Thioridazine		to void
Opiate analgesics		
Diamorphine,	Pain control, drug	Bladder sphincter spasm
morphine	abuse	causing difficulty in
		micturition and urge urinary
		incontinence
Xanthines		
Theophylline	Asthma	Increased diuresis, aggravates
Caffeine		detrusor overactivity causing
		urge urinary incontinence

MEDICATION WHICH REDUCES THE SIZE OF THE PROSTATE GLAND

Drug therapy using 5-alpha reductase inhibitors decreases the size of the prostate by inhibiting the enzyme necessary for testosterone metabolism. Finasteride (Proscar) and dutasteride (Avodart) are 5-alpha reductase inhibitors which are used to treat urethral blockage from benign prostate hypertrophy. Dutasteride produces symptomatic responses in approximately 3 months whilst finasteride takes approximately 6 months. Flow rate improvements and prostate volume changes are seen at approximately 1 month with dutasteride. If the medication is withdrawn, the prostate gland will return to pretreatment size or rebound with an increase in size. Finasteride and dutasteride act by androgen deprivation and may be responsible for loss of libido in some men.

Serenoa repens, an extract from the berries of the American dwarf saw palmetto plant, is used to block 5-alpha reductase, thereby reducing the size of the prostate gland. From a systematic review of 18 randomised controlled trials, evidence suggested that serenoa repens improved urologic symptoms and urinary flow (Wilt et al. 1998). When compared to finasteride, serenoa repens produced similar improvement in lower urinary tract symptoms with fewer adverse effects. However, the long-term effectiveness remains unknown.

MEDICATION WHICH RELAXES THE SMOOTH MUSCLE OF THE BLADDER NECK

Alpha-adrenoreceptor antagonists (Tamulosin, Alfuzosin, Doxazosin) (Hytrin in the USA) are uroselective alpha-blockers which can be used for symptoms of obstruction owing to their relaxant effect on the prostate smooth muscle and internal urethral sphincter. These medications increase urinary flow and decrease frequency and have fewer side-effects than prazosin hydrochloride (Hypovaze) and doxazosin mesylate (Cardura). However, alpha-blockers may also have an effect on the intestinal smooth muscle resulting in constipation. Patients are warned they may have retrograde ejaculation. These alpha-blockers may cause side-effects of dry mouth, sedation, dizziness, drowsiness, tachycardia and palpitations.

MEDICATION FOR PROSTATE CANCER

Endocrine therapy includes gonadotrophin-releasing hormone antagonists (GnRHas) such as goserelin (Zoladex), leuprorelin (Prostap) and decapeptyl (Triptorelin). Anti-androgen drug treatment such as cyproterone acetate and bicalutamide (Casodex) is used as a treatment for prostate cancer. Side-effects include gynaecomastia, loss of libido and erectile dysfunction.

MEDICATION FOR HYPOCONTRACTILE BLADDER

Cholinergic agonists such as Carbachol and Bethanechol can enhance detrusor contractions during micturition, provided the problem is not too severe. Their use is limited owing to lack of efficacy.

MEDICATION FOR ERECTILE DYSFUNCTION

Medication for erectile dysfunction is reported in Chapter 15.

MEDICATION WHICH CHANGES THE COLOUR OF THE URINE

Urine is a natural waste product of the body which is typically clear and pale to deep yellow in colour owing to the pigment urochrome which is derived from the body's destruction of haemoglobin. As urine becomes more concentrated, it becomes deeper yellow, although changes in colour may reflect diet or medication, or may be due to blood or bile in the urine. Colour, as well as taste and smell, of the urine can be an indication of the patient's condition. Ford (1992) described a range of substances or conditions which coloured urine:

Red	Phenytoin, senna, beetroot, blackberries, heamaturia, nephritis
Orange	Warfarin, rifampicillin, paprika, rhubarb, dehydration
Yellow	Nitrofurantoin, sulphonamides, vitamins, asparagus
Green	Amitriptyline, indomethacin, jaundice, urine infection
Blue	Amitriptyline, triamterene, typhus
Purple	Phenolphthalein, senna, high-protein diet porphyria
Brown	Iron preparations, metronidazole, liver and gall bladder disease
Black	Methyldopa, quinine, malignant melanoma

SUMMARY

Medication may be used in conjunction with physical therapy for a number of urological conditions such as detrusor overactivity, nocturnal enuresis, nocturia and benign prostatic hyperplasia.

Antimuscarinic drug therapy may be prescribed for moderate and severe detrusor overactivity. Antidiuretic hormone analogues may be prescribed for nocturnal enuresis. Drug therapy using 5-alpha reductase inhibitors reduces the size of the prostate, while alpha-blockers relax the smooth muscle of the bladder neck.

Endocrine therapy or anti-androgen drug treatment may be prescribed for prostate cancer.

Certain groups of drugs such as diuretics, calcium-channel antagonists, non-steroidal anti-inflammatory drugs, sedative medication, sleeping tablets and anticholinergics may have an adverse effect on lower urinary tract function, especially in the elderly.

13 Faecal Incontinence

Key points

- Faecal leakage may be related to evacuation dysfunction, constipation, functional disability, impaired consciousness, neurological conditions, bowel urgency and diarrhoea.
- Treatment is multifactorial and may include diet, avoiding constipation, defaecation advice, relaxation and pelvic floor muscle exercises.

INTRODUCTION

In normal digestion, waste products called faeces are stored in the rectum in preparation for elimination from the body in a process called defaecation. Occasionally faecal leakage occurs; it can be due to a number of factors.

DIGESTIVE SYSTEM

Food and drink enters the mouth, mixes with saliva and travels through the oesophagus to the stomach where it is stored and digested with the help of enzymes. When digestion is completed, the stomach pumps the food into the duodenum. Bile from the gall bladder travels through the bile duct into the duodenum to break down fat. Food is moved along the gut by involuntary waves of muscle contraction called peristalsis. In the small intestine, food nutrients and vitamins are absorbed into the blood stream. In the large intestine, water is absorbed and the faeces are prepared for defaecation. Faeces are stored in the rectum prior to expulsion through the anus. (See Figure 13.1.)

There are three controlling sphincters in the digestive tract, which are under involuntary control. The gastric sphincter prevents food in the stomach from regurgitating back into the oesophagus. The duodenal sphincter prevents food from entering the small intestine until it has been properly digested in the stomach. The internal anal sphincter automatically prevents the faeces from entering the anus until there is an appropriate time and place to defaecate. The external anal sphincter and pelvic floor muscles are under voluntary control and reinforce the action of the internal anal sphincter.

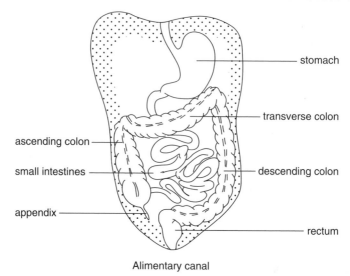

Figure 13.1. Alimentary canal (Reproduced by permission of NEEN Mobilis Healthcare Group. *Source*: Dorey, 2004b)

DEFAECATION

The rectum lies in front of the sacrum. The rectum joins the anal canal at the anorectal junction where it is surrounded by the pelvic floor muscles. The anus is about 4 cm long in men and has an involuntary circular internal anal sphincter which is surrounded by a circular voluntary external anal sphincter. The external anal sphincter connects above with the deep pelvic floor muscles and in front to the other superficial pelvic floor muscles. (See Figures 13.2 and 13.3.)

Bowel patterns may vary from 1–3 times a day to once in 3 days. Usually, faeces are expelled following a reflex contraction of the digestive tract after eating or having a warm drink at breakfast time. When passing a bowel motion, the external anal sphincter and pelvic floor muscles relax, the diaphragm pushes downwards and the abdominal muscles brace and bulge to expel the faeces.

PELVIC FLOOR MUSCLES

The pelvic floor muscles form a muscular shelf across the bottom of the pelvis. Tightening the pelvic floor muscles helps to contain urine, faeces and flatus within the body until the time and place are convenient for elimination. The

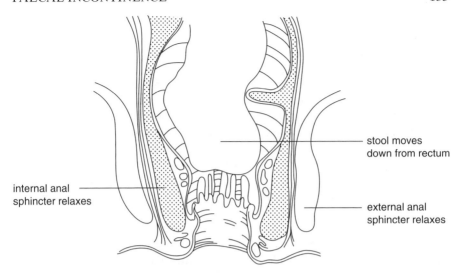

stool moves
down from rectum

internal anal
sphincter relaxes

external anal
sphincter relaxes

Figure 13.2. Defaecation (Reproduced by permission of NEEN Mobilis Healthcare Group. *Source*: Dorey, 2004b)

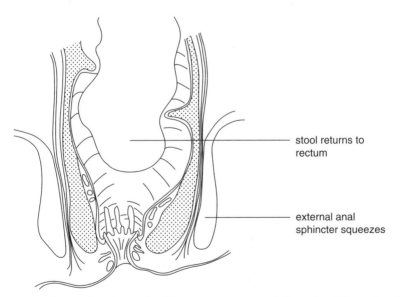

stool returns to
rectum

external anal
sphincter squeezes

Figure 13.3. Squeezing the anal sphincter to postpone defaecation (Reproduced by permission of NEEN Mobilis Healthcare Group. *Source*: Dorey, 2004b)

puborectalis muscle maintains the anorectal angle and helps to stop faeces from entering the anal canal.

The male pelvic floor muscles are subject to fatigue, stretching and injury. Events such as prostate surgery, abdominal surgery, sexual abuse, obesity, constipation, persistent coughing, lifting, pushing, prolonged standing, cycling, pelvic injury and ageing may affect the normal function of the pelvic floor muscles. Men may sustain neurological damage during treatment for prostate cancer, such as radical prostatectomy and radiotherapy. Neurological conditions such as multiple sclerosis, spinal cord injury, stroke and Parkinson's disease may compromise the nerves which serve the external anal sphincter and the pelvic floor muscles. Occasionally both internal and external anal sphincters may be damaged during anal surgery for haemorrhoids or anal fissures.

Rectal prolapse (Figure 13.4) occurs when the ligaments holding the rectum in place become weakened, allowing the rectal wall to descend and prolapse through the anus. If the prolapse does not return back within the body after voiding faeces, surgery may be indicated.

A weak pelvic floor may be unable to withstand the gravitational and intra-abdominal forces of jumping, resulting in urinary and faecal leakage. Smoking makes all the involuntary muscle in the body contract and may contribute to faecal urgency. Repeated coughing places extra strain on the pelvic floor. Excess weight, constipation and heavy or repeated lifting also places extra strain on the pelvic floor.

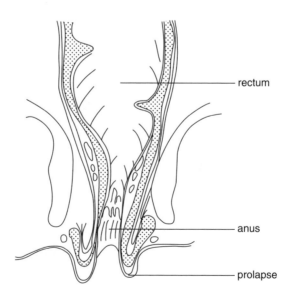

rectum

anus

prolapse

Figure 13.4. Rectal prolapse (Reproduced by permission of NEEN Mobilis Health-care Group. *Source*: Dorey, 2004b)

As men age, the pelvic floor muscles may weaken if regular pelvic floor exercises are not performed.

CAUSES OF FAECAL LEAKAGE

There are several types of faecal incontinence (Potter et al. 2002). Faecal leakage may be related to evacuation dysfunction, constipation, functional disability, impaired consciousness, neurological conditions, faecal urgency and diarrhoea.

FAECAL LEAKAGE RELATED TO EVACUATION DYSFUNCTION

Evacuation dysfunction occurs when men contract rather than relax the puborectalis muscle, external anal sphincter and surrounding muscles whilst trying to defaecate. Anxiety can produce hypertonus and usually makes the problem worse. Evacuation dysfunction can lead to constipation and overflow incontinence of fluid faecal matter and mucus. Evacuation dysfunction also occurs when men are unable or unwilling to generate an adequate abdominal expulsive force.

FAECAL LEAKAGE RELATED TO CONSTIPATION

Faecal leakage may be caused by severe constipation causing fluid faecal matter and mucus to overflow and leak. This type of faecal leakage is also called overflow incontinence.

CONSTIPATION

Constipation may be defined as the infrequent passage of hard stool, excessive straining when trying to defaecate, and a feeling of incomplete emptying. Constipation may be caused by a slow propulsion of waste products through the colon and the inability to know when the rectum is full and needs emptying. Certain medications delay the propulsion of waste products through the colon. Constipation may be self-induced by ignoring a call to void faeces owing to a busy lifestyle or by a reluctance to use the toilet when not at home. Pain from an anal fissure or from haemorrhoids may lead to constipation and may require appropriate surgery. The elderly are more likely to develop constipation, particularly those taking more than five medications a day and those taking anticholinergic drugs, diuretics, beta-blockers, antidepressants, asthma medication or tranquillisers. Other risk factors which contribute to constipation are: a sedentary lifestyle, particularly those in nursing homes, those with Parkinson's disease, diabetes mellitus, spinal cord injury, stroke, dehydration, dementia and depression (Potter et al. 2002). A greatly enlarged prostate can contribute to constipation.

FAECAL LEAKAGE RELATED TO FUNCTIONAL DISABILITY

Poor mobility, poor dexterity and poor vision may make it difficult for some people to reach the toilet in time resulting in faecal leakage.

FAECAL LEAKAGE DUE TO IMPAIRED CONSCIOUSNESS

Men and women with dementia, impaired consciousness and behavioural problems may be unaware of a need to evacuate their bowel and may experience faecal leakage.

FAECAL LEAKAGE RELATED TO NEUROLOGICAL CONDITIONS

Neurological conditions in which the nerves to the colon and pelvic floor muscles are damaged may contribute to faecal incontinence.

FAECAL LEAKAGE RELATED TO FAECAL URGENCY

Faecal urge incontinence occurs following a strong urge to empty the bowels. If the internal anal sphincter is damaged, passive soiling may occur. If the external anal sphincter and the pelvic floor muscles are weak or unable to contract, faecal leakage may occur on the way to the bathroom. Damage to the anal sphincter may be due to anal surgery, anal stretch, previous surgery, chronic straining to pass faeces or sexual abuse.

FAECAL INCONTINENCE RELATED TO DIARRHOEA

Faecal leakage may be caused by the inability to hold diarrhoea. Diarrhoea can be caused by infection, medication side-effect, laxative abuse, irritable bowel syndrome, inflammatory bowel disease, bowel cancer, bowel surgery, radiotherapy and anxiety.

TREATMENT FOR FAECAL LEAKAGE
ASSESSMENT

Men may be referred for treatment by their urologist, colorectal surgeon or GP, or they may self-refer. A detailed assessment by a specialist continence physiotherapist or continence nurse specialist must be undertaken so that appropriate treatment can be provided. The therapist will explain the problem with the help of diagrams and/or a model of the pelvic floor muscles. Following informed consent, the therapist will perform a gentle anal examination to assess the strength, endurance and integrity of the pelvic floor muscles. The correct exercise programme can then be 'tailor-made' to each individual. If physiotherapy is not the desired treatment, patients will be referred on to the most appropriate professional.

TREATMENT FOR EVACUATION DYSFUNCTION

Those men with evacuation dysfunction due to pelvic floor muscle hypertonus may be treated with biofeedback and relaxation techniques. Men should be taught how to bear down and relax the anal sphincter and pelvic floor muscles during voiding faeces.

Men who do not generate sufficient pressure to void may be taught how to sit well on the toilet. Defaecation is easier when using a good functional position. Men should lean forwards with the knees higher than the hips and the hands or elbows on the thighs. During attempted defaecation they should breathe normally and allow the external anal sphincter and pelvic floor muscles to relax whilst the diaphragm pushes down and the abdominal muscles bulge out forwards and sideways. Men should not strain.

TREATMENT FOR CONSTIPATION

The consistency of faeces varies from day to day according to the type of food eaten, quantity of fluid drunk, level of exercise taken and level of stress experienced (Table 13.1). Hard pellet stools are more common in slow transit constipation. Loose stools increase the possibility of suffering from passive faecal leakage and faecal urge incontinence. Optimum stool firmness would be Type 3 or Type 4 on the Bristol Stool Form Scale (Figure 13.5). Certain foods make the stool more solid whilst some foods make the stool softer and

Table 13.1. How to avoid constipation

Review existing medication
Eat a healthy diet with plenty of fruit and green vegetables daily
Have cultured yoghurt daily
Drink 1½ litres of fluid a day
Avoid an excess of alcoholic drinks
Eat breakfast
Never ignore a call to pass a motion
Make time to visit the bathroom before rushing off to work
Improve access to toilet
Avoid sitting for long periods
Sit in a good position on the toilet
After voiding faeces, tighten your anal sphincter before wiping your bottom
Avoid enemas and laxatives, which may cause constipation after use

If men are severely constipated they should visit their GP or practice nurse

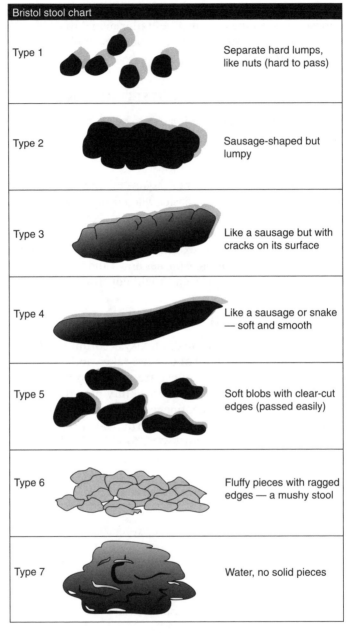

Figure 13.5. Bristol Stool Form Scale (Reproduced by permission of Dr K Heaton and NEEN Mobilis Healthcare Group. *Source*: O'Donnell et al., 1990)

easier to pass. Fibre helps the stool to retain water and makes it softer and easier to pass (Table 13.2).

TREATMENT FOR FAECAL OVERFLOW INCONTINENCE

Faecal leakage may be caused by severe constipation causing fluid faecal matter to overflow and leak. Constipation may be avoided by maintaining a regular balanced diet containing fibre products.

It is not always advisable to increase dietary fibre if constipation already exists as this may increase faecal loading and increase the risk of faecal incontinence. It may be necessary to use prescribed mild laxatives to soften the stool. It is important to make sure men have audio and visual privacy when using the toilet.

TREATMENT FOR FAECAL INCONTINENCE DUE TO FUNCTIONAL DISABILITY

Physiotherapy and occupational therapy may help men with poor mobility and poor dexterity. Men may be advised to wear clothes that are easy to unfasten and have easy access to the toilet or have a commode close at hand.

Table 13.2. Effect of different foods on stool formation

EXAMPLES OF FOODS WHICH MAKE THE STOOL FIRMER

Meat
Eggs
Hard cheese
White bread

EXAMPLES OF FOODS WHICH MAKE THE STOOL SOFTER

Green vegetables
Beans
Salad
Fruit
High-fibre cereals
Wholemeal bread and biscuits
Nuts

FOOD WHICH MAY PRODUCE WIND

Beans, peas and pulses
Onions and leeks
Cabbage and cauliflower
Peanuts
Cucumber
Sultanas
Artichokes (both globe and Jerusalem)

TREATMENT FOR FAECAL INCONTINENCE DUE TO IMPAIRED CONSCIOUSNESS

Men with faecal leakage due to impaired consciousness should be referred to the continence advisor for the correct type and size of pads.

TREATMENT FOR FAECAL INCONTINENCE DUE TO NEUROLOGICAL CONDITIONS

Men with faecal leakage due to mild or moderate neurological impairment may be helped with pelvic floor muscle exercises, voiding advice and attention to diet. For men with normal or partial neurological control of the pelvic floor muscles, the external anal sphincter and the pelvic floor muscles should be strengthened. Muscle endurance can be increased by lifting the pelvic floor muscles about 50 % of maximum whilst walking and can be used following an urge to void faeces. Voiding advice consists of good toilet positioning and gaining the feeling of relaxing the pelvic floor muscles during voiding. Biofeedback is a useful adjunct to relaxation for men with voiding dysfunction.

Men with severe neurological deficit should be referred to the continence advisor for the correct type and size of pads. Surgery may be indicated (see opposite).

TREATMENT FOR FAECAL URGENCY

The external anal sphincter and the pelvic floor muscles should be strengthened to prevent faecal leakage following an urge to pass a motion. Men with faecal urge incontinence should tighten the pelvic floor muscles about 50 % of maximum whilst walking to the bathroom to prevent faecal leakage.

It may be prudent to cut down on foods such as onions, curries, chillis and caffeine products which stimulate the smooth muscle of the gut and can make faecal urgency worse.

TREATMENT FOR DIARRHOEA

Men and women with prolonged diarrhoea should visit the GP, who will assess each patient individually. The GP will review medication and laxatives, and may conduct further tests for infection and bowel disease.

ADVICE FOR MEN WITH FAECAL INCONTINENCE

Table 13.3 gives detailed advice and lifestyle guidance for men with faecal incontinence.

After voiding faeces, men should tighten their anal sphincter before wiping their bottom. This returns the faeces not voided back up to the rectum above the anorectal junction.

Table 13.3. Advice for men with faecal incontinence

Perform pelvic floor muscle exercises daily
Tighten pelvic floor muscles during coughing, sneezing and lifting
Watch weight to avoid overloading your pelvic floor
Eat a balanced diet
Drink 1½ litres of fluid a day
Eat breakfast
Make time to visit the toilet after breakfast
Tighten pelvic floor muscles on way to bathroom
Tighten pelvic floor muscles after voiding faeces
Avoid a sedentary lifestyle

Visit GP if men experience:
    Fresh blood or dark red blood in faeces
    Severe constipation
    Abdominal pain
    Continual diarrhoea
    Unexplained change in bowel habit
    Severe bowel problems preventing men from leaving home

The local continence advisor will advise men with severe or regular leakage about the appropriate shape and style of pad. Men may need help with skin care and odour control. Some pads are free of charge within the NHS. An anal plug may be considered in selected situations.

SURGERY

There are a number of surgical options for men who suffer from severe faecal incontinence. A colorectal surgeon will discuss which options are best for each patient. Surgery is best performed at a specialist hospital which performs a large number of similar operations. Post-surgical complications include infection.

Anal sphincter repair may be indicated for patients who have experienced disruption of the external anal sphincter as a result of trauma or following surgery for anal fistula repair. This operation may result in satisfactory long-term anal continence in 50 % of cases (Morren et al. 2001). It is rarely performed in the UK.

Graciloplasty is an operation where a thigh muscle is used to encircle the anal sphincter. The muscle is stimulated through electrodes implanted close to the nerve which are attached to a neurostimulator implanted under the abdominal wall. Satisfactory anal continence has been reported in 50–73 % of cases (Christiansen et al. 1998). It is rarely performed in the UK.

Artificial anal sphincter is surgery in which an inflatable cuff is implanted around the anal canal and connected to a reservoir in the abdomen. A control pump is placed in the scrotum. Results from this operation are encouraging (Christiansen et al. 1999).

Sacral nerve stimulation is a comparatively new form of surgery in which the sacral nerves are stimulated through electrodes implanted into the sacrum. These are attached to a stimulator implanted under the buttock.

Occasionally, a colostomy may be performed for men without bowel control. The colon is brought to the surface of the abdomen and the faeces collected in a discreet bag. Patients may find that the quality of life with a stoma appliance is more socially acceptable than life coping with severe uncontrolled faecal incontinence. Patient care is provided by stoma nurses.

SUMMARY

Faecal leakage may be related to evacuation dysfunction, constipation, functional disability, impaired consciousness, neurological conditions, faecal urgency and diarrhoea. Treatment is multifactorial and may include advice concerning diet, avoiding constipation, defaecation advice, relaxation and pelvic floor muscle exercises.

14 Male Sexual Dysfunction

Key points

- Male sexual function is dependent on satisfactory libido, erectile function, orgasm and ejaculation.
- Sexual dysfunction occurs when there is a problem with any of these.
- Erectile dysfunction is a common condition which is strongly age-related.
- Pelvic floor muscles are active during penile erection and ejaculation.

INTRODUCTION

Sexual function in healthy men is dependent on satisfactory libido, erectile function, orgasm and ejaculation. Sexual dysfunction occurs when there is a problem with any of these. Sexual dysfunction embraces low libido, erectile dysfunction, premature ejaculation, retrograde ejaculation, retarded ejaculation, anorgasmia, anejaculation, aspermia, haemospermia, low-volume ejaculate, painful ejaculation, anhedonia and sexual pain.

LOW LIBIDO

DEFINITION

A low libido can be defined as 'a reduced sexual urge'. As men age, there is a gradual partial androgen decline.

CLASSIFICATION OF DIFFERENT FORMS

Men can be classified as having low or absent libido.

PREVALENCE

The exact prevalence of men who have low libido remains unknown. It is estimated that at 40 years of age, there will be a 10 % decline of total testosterone every decade, although the mechanisms are not fully understood (1st Latin American Erectile Dysfunction Consensus Meeting, 2003a).

AETIOLOGY

The cause of diminished libido is as a result of ageing and a gradual decline in androgen production. The testis produces 95–98 % of androgren production with the adrenal glands producing the remaining 2–5 % (1st Latin American Erectile Dysfunction Consensus Meeting, 2003a).

ERECTILE DYSFUNCTION

Erectile dysfunction is a common condition which is linked to increasing age and age-related diseases. Men with erectile dysfunction suffer from depression and low self-esteem, and experience difficulties establishing and maintaining relationships.

DEFINITION

Erectile dysfunction is defined as 'the inability to achieve or maintain an erection sufficient for satisfactory sexual performance (for both partners)' (National Institutes of Health Consensus Development Panel on Impotence, 1993).

CLASSIFICATION OF DIFFERENT FORMS

The severity of erectile dysfunction has been classified as mild, moderate or severe. Men who achieve satisfactory sexual performance in 7 to 8 attempts out of 10 are classified as having mild erectile dysfunction; those who achieve 4 to 6 out of 10 are classified moderate; and those who achieve 0 to 3 out of 10 are classified severe. (Albaugh & Lewis 1999.)

PREVALENCE

The exact prevalence of erectile dysfunction is unknown. An estimated 152 million men worldwide suffered from erectile dysfunction in 1995 and this figure was projected to rise to 322 million men worldwide in 2025 (Aytac et al. 1999). It is a common problem and strongly age-related (Feldman et al. 1994). Erectile dysfunction affects more than 20 % of men under 40 years of age, more than 50 % of men over 40 years of age and more than 66 % of men over 70 years of age (Feldman et al. 1994; Heruti et al. 2004). It may affect 10 % of healthy men and significantly greater numbers of men with existing co-morbidities such as hypertension (15 %), diabetes (28 %) and heart disease (39 %) (Wagner et al. 1996; Feldman et al. 1994). The number of men is predicted to rise with increased life expectancy and a growing population of elderly people.

AETIOLOGY

The causes of erectile dysfunction are listed in Table 14.1.

Risk factors for erectile dysfunction include vascular insufficiency, hormonal abnormalities, interruption of the neural pathways and psychogenic factors (Feldman et al. 1994).

Also, Lewis and Mills (1999) listed 332 prescription drugs that have been associated with erectile dysfunction. These include psychotrophic drugs, cardiovascular drugs, histamine-2-receptor antagonists, hormones, anticholinergics and certain cytotoxic agents. Another risk factor is diabetes mellitus, where as many as 50 % of men may suffer from erectile dysfunction (Benet & Melman 1995).

Weak pelvic floor muscles compromise penile erection (Colpi et al. 1999; Dorey et al. 2004a).

Other risk factors include accidental trauma, trauma from surgery and radiation therapy. Lifestyle-related factors include cigarette-smoking, chronic obstructive lung disease, alcohol abuse, drug abuse, bicycling and horse-riding.

PSYCHOLOGICAL CAUSES

Erectile dysfunction always has a psychological component in addition to the underlying cause (Intili & Nier 1998). In a pilot study of 15 men Intili and Nier (1998) found a link between erectile dysfunction and both depression and low self-esteem.

The psychological causes of erectile dysfunction have been classified as: religious orthodoxy, obsessive-compulsive personality, gender identity, sexual phobias, widower's syndrome, fear of pregnancy, marital conflict, depression, lack of attraction to partner, fear of closeness, poor body image and concern over ageing (LoPiccolo 1986). However, the International Society of Impotence Research (ISIR) divides psychogenic factors into 'Generalised Type', which includes 'Generalised unresponsiveness' and 'Generalised inhibition', and 'Situational Type', which includes 'Partner related', 'Performance related' and 'Psychological distress or adjustment related' (Lizza & Rosen 1999) (Table 14.2).

ANATOMY OF THE PENIS

The internal structure of the penis consists of three cylindrical bodies: dorsally, the two corpora cavernosa communicate with each other for three-quarters of their length and ventrally the corpus spongiosum surrounds the penile portion of the urethra (Figure 14.1). The proximal end of the corpus spongiosum forms a bulb attached to the urogenital diaphragm and at the

Table 14.1. Risk factors for erectile dysfunction

Risk factor	Possible components	Reference
Psychogenic	Marital conflict Depression Poor body image Performance-related Bereavement	Feldman et al. (1994)
Vasculogenic	Arteriogenic Venogenic Ischaemia	Feldman et al. (1994) Feldman et al. (1994) Berger et al. (2005)
Neurogenic	Spinal cord trauma Multiple sclerosis Spinal tumours Parkinson's disease	Feldman et al. (1994)
Endocrinologic	Hormonal deficiency	Feldman et al. (1994)
Diabetic	Peripheral neuropathy Hypertension Renal failure	Benet & Melman (1995)
Drug-related	Some antihypertensives Some psychotropics Hormonal agents	Benet & Melman (1995)
Surgical trauma	Transurethral and radical prostatectomy Pelvic surgery Radiotherapy	Lewis & Mills (1999)

Lower urinary
    tract symptoms
	Severity of lower urinary
	    tract symptoms,
	    particularly incontinence
		Frankel et al. (1998)

Prostatic	Benign prostatic hyperplasia	Baniel et al. (2000)
Lifestyle-related	Trauma to the perineum Bicycling Nicotine abuse Drug abuse Alcohol abuse	Bortolotti et al. (1997) Andersen & Bovim (1997) Rosen et al. (1991) Lewis & Mills (1999) Fabra & Porst (1999)
Weak pelvic floor musculature	Weak pelvic floor muscles Ageing	Dorey et al. (2004a) Colpi et al. (1999)

Table 14.2. Classification of the psychological causes of erectile dysfunction (Reproduced by permission of John Wiley & Sons. *Source*: Dorey, 2001b)

LoPiccolo (LoPiccolo 1986)	ISIR classification (Lizza & Rosen 1999)
Psychological causes	*Psychogenic factors*
Religious orthodoxy	*Generalised type:*
Obsessive-compulsive personality	Generalised unresponsiveness
Gender identity	Generalised inhibition
Sexual phobias	
Widower's syndrome	*Situational type:*
Fear of pregnancy	Partner related
Marital conflict	Performance related
Depression	Psychological distress or
Lack of attraction to partner	Adjustment related
Fear of closeness	
Poor body image	
Concern over ageing	

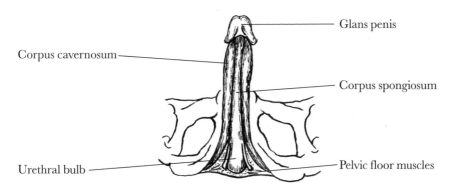

Figure 14.1. Anatomy of the penis (Reproduced by permission of John Wiley & Sons. *Source*: Dorey, 2001b)

distal end expands to form the glans penis (Kirby et al. 1999). The tunica albuginea, which is composed of two layers of elastic and collagen fibres, surrounds the erectile bodies.

The erectile tissue in the corpora cavernosa and the corpus spongiosum comprises vascular lacunar spaces, which are surrounded by smooth muscle (Figure 14.2). The lacunar spaces derive blood from the helicine arteries, which open directly into these sinusoids. Subtunical veins between the inner and outer tunica albuginea form a network and drain blood from the erectile tissue.

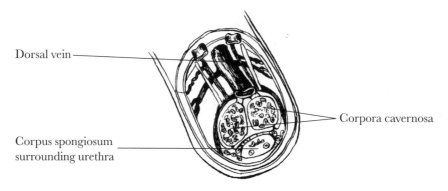

Figure 14.2. Cross-section of the penis (Reproduced by permission of John Wiley & Sons. *Source*: Dorey, 2001b)

NEUROPHYSIOLOGY OF PENILE ERECTION

From a neurophysiological aspect, erection can be classified into three types (Brock & Lue 1993):

(1) Reflexogenic erection

Reflexogenic erection originates from tactile stimulation to the genitalia. Impulses reach the spinal erection centre via sacral sensory nerves (S2–4) and thoracic nerves (T10–L2) and some follow the ascending tract culminating in sensory perception, while others activate the autonomic nuclei of the efferent nerves which induce the erection process.

(2) Psychogenic erection

Psychogenic erection originates from audiovisual stimuli or fantasy. Signals descend to the spinal erection centre to activate the erection process.

(3) Nocturnal erection

Nocturnal erection occurs mostly during the rapid eye movement stage of sleep. Most men experience three to five erections lasting up to 30 minutes in a normal night's sleep (Fisher et al. 1965). Central impulses descend the spinal cord (through an unknown mechanism) to activate the erection process.

PATHOPHYSIOLOGY OF PENILE ERECTION

Penile erection occurs following a series of integrated vascular processes culminating in the accumulation of blood under pressure and end-organ rigidity (Moncada Iribarren & Sáenz de Tejada 1999). This vascular process can be divided into six phases:

(1) Flaccidity

A state of low flow of blood and low pressure exists in the penis in the flaccid state (Figure 14.3). The ischiocavernosus and bulbocavernosus muscles are relaxed.

(2) Filling phase

When the erection mechanism is initiated, the parasympathetic nervous system provides excitory input to the penis from efferent segments S2–4 of the sacral spinal cord, the penile smooth arterial muscle relaxes and the

Flaccid state

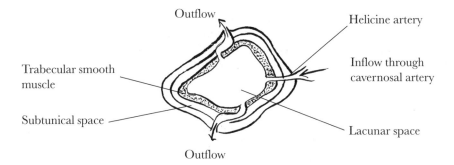

Erect State

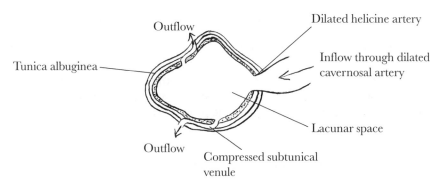

Figure 14.3. Veno-occlusive mechanism of penile erection (Reproduced by permission of John Wiley & Sons. *Source*: Dorey, 2001b)

cavernosal and helicine arteries dilate enabling blood to flow into the lacunar spaces.

(3) Tumescence

The venous outflow is reduced by the compression of the subtunical venules against the tunica albuginea (corporal veno-occlusive mechanism) causing the penis to expand and elongate but with a scant increase in intracavernous pressure.

(4) Full erection

The intracavernous pressure rapidly increases to produce full penile erection.

(5) Rigidity

The intracavernous pressure rises above the diastolic pressure and blood inflow occurs with the systolic phase of the pulse enabling complete rigidity to occur. Contraction or reflex contraction of the ischiocavernosus and bulbocavernosus muscles produces changes in the intracavernous pressure. When full rigidity is achieved, no further arterial flow occurs (Figure 14.3).

(6) Detumescence

The sympathetic nervous system is responsible for detumescence via thoracolumbar segments (T10–12, L1–2) in the spinal cord. Contraction of the smooth muscles of the penis and contraction of the penile arteries lead to a decrease of blood in the lacunar spaces and the contraction of the smooth trabecular muscle leads to a collapse of the lacunar spaces and detumescence.

PATHOPHYSIOLOGY OF ERECTILE DYSFUNCTION

Three types of erectile dysfunction are acknowledged: psychogenic, organic and mixed. They may be primary or secondary after a period of normal erectile function (1st Latin American Erectile Dysfunction Consensus Meeting, 2003b). In organic erectile dysfunction, the events leading to full erection fail to occur owing to insufficient blood reaching the penis or owing to blood escaping from the penis.

ROLE OF THE PELVIC FLOOR MUSCLES

The ischiocavernosus and bulbocavernosus muscles (Figure 14.4) are active during penile erection. Contractions of the ischiocavernosus muscles produce

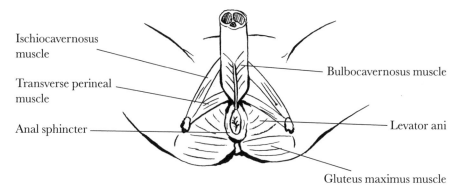

Ischiocavernosus muscle

Transverse perineal muscle

Anal sphincter

Bulbocavernosus muscle

Levator ani

Gluteus maximus muscle

Figure 14.4. Male superficial pelvic floor muscles (Reproduced by permission of John Wiley & Sons. *Source*: Dorey, 2001b)

an increase in the intracavernous pressure and influence penile rigidity. The area of the corpora cavernosum compressed by the ischiocavernosus muscle ranges from 35.6% to 55.9% (Claes et al. 1996). The middle fibres of the bulbocavernosus muscle assist in erection of the corpus spongiosum penis by compressing the erectile tissue of the bulb of the penis. The anterior fibres spread out over the side of the corpus cavernosum and are attached to the fascia covering the dorsal vessels of the penis and contribute to erection by compressing the deep dorsal vein of the penis thus preventing the outflow of blood from the penis.

Weak pelvic floor muscles compromise penile erection (Colpi et al. 1999; Dorey et al. 2004a).

ORGASMIC AND EJACULATORY DISORDERS

The final phase of sexual response in men culminates in orgasm and ejaculation. Although erection and ejaculation are co-ordinated, they are produced by different mechanisms.

CLASSIFICATION OF DIFFERENT FORMS

Orgasmic and ejaculatory disorders may be classified as anorgasmia, anejaculation, premature ejaculation, retrograde ejaculation and delayed ejaculation, aspermia, haemospermia, low-volume ejaculate, painful ejaculation and anhedonia (Ralph & Wylie 2005). Ejaculatory disorders such as anejaculation, delayed ejaculation and premature ejaculation may lead to complete or partial loss of the ejaculate needed for impregnation of the female partner.

ANORGASMIA

DEFINITION

Anorgasmia is defined as 'the inability to achieve orgasm during conscious sexual activity, although nocturnal emission may occur' (Hendry et al. 2000).

CLASSIFICATION OF DIFFERENT FORMS

Anorgasmia may be congenital, acquired and/or psychological (Hendry 1999).

PREVALENCE

The exact prevalence of anorgasmia is unknown. However, 37% of men post radical prostatectomy reported anorgasmia, and a further 37% reported a decreased intensity of orgasm (Barnas et al. 2004).

AETIOLOGY

There are a number of causes of anorgasmia. These range from congenital abnormalities, surgical trauma following imperforate anus, para-aortic lymphadenectomy or prostate surgery, genital infections such as gonorrhoea or nonspecific urethritis, spinal cord injury, antidepressants, antipsychotics and polycystic kidney associated with dilatation of the seminal vesicles (Hendry 1999).

ANEJACULATION

DEFINITION

Anejaculation is defined as 'the absence of ejaculation during orgasm' (Hendry et al. 2000).

CLASSIFICATION OF DIFFERENT FORMS

Anejaculation may be congenital or acquired and/or psychological (1st Latin American Erectile Dysfunction Consensus Meeting, 2003c).

PREVALENCE

The prevalence of anejaculation is unknown.

MECHANISM OF EJACULATION

Stimulation of the superior hypogastric or hypogastric nerves causes contraction of the bladder neck, seminal vesicles and ejaculatory ducts resulting in ejaculation. Ejaculation comprises a sympathetic phase followed by a somatic phase (Ralph & Wylie 2005). It can occur independently of penile erection. The sympathetically mediated emission of seminal fluid into the posterior urethra is followed by a somatically mediated true ejaculation with expulsion of the ejaculate. Sympathetic efferent fibres from the hypogastric nerve (T10–L2) cause sequential contraction of the epididymus, vas deferens, seminal vesicles and prostate with closure of the bladder neck. True ejaculation is then mediated via the pudendal nerve (S2–4) causing rhythmical contractions of the bulbocavernosus muscles which force the ejaculate through the distal urethra. There is contraction of the periurethral and pelvic floor muscles combined with intermittent relaxation of the external urinary sphincter and urogenital diaphragm to allow ejaculation (Krane et al. 1989). The experience of orgasm is independent of sympathetic and parasympathetic activity but it does require an intact pudendal nerve (Mamberti-Dias et al. 1999).

AETIOLOGY

Ejaculatory dysfunction can be due to congenital abnormalities, surgical trauma, genital infection, stones in the ejaculatory duct, paraplegia or dilatation of the seminal vesicles, or it can be functional (Hendry et al. 2000). Functional ejaculatory dysfunction includes congenital anorgasmia, where an overstrict upbringing may produce an inability to achieve orgasm, premature ejaculation and the side-effects of some antihypertensive and psychotropic drugs.

RETROGRADE EJACULATION

DEFINITION

Retrograde ejaculation is defined as 'backward passage of semen into the bladder after emission usually due to failure of closure of the bladder neck mechanism, demonstrated by presence of spermatozoa in the urine after orgasm' (Hendry et al. 2000).

CLASSIFICATION OF DIFFERENT FORMS

Retrograde ejaculation can be congenital or acquired and/or psychological (1st Latin American Erectile Dysfunction Consensus Meeting, 2003c).

PREVALENCE

Retrograde ejaculation occurs in 75 % of men after transurethral resection of prostate and, to a lesser extent, after bladder neck incision (Dunsmuir et al. 1996).

AETIOLOGY

Retrograde ejaculation can be due to damage of the bladder neck during prostate surgery, bladder neck disorder from alpha-adrenergic, neuroleptic or antidepressant blocking agents, diabetes, and some neuropathies (1st Latin American Erectile Dysfunction Consensus Meeting, 2003c).

RETARDED EJACULATION

Retarded ejaculation is defined as 'undue delay in reaching a climax during sexual activity' (Hendry et al. 2000).

PREVALENCE

The prevalence of retarded ejaculation and orgasmic disorders is 2.5 % in patients with sexual problems attending their GP (Nazareth et al. 2003). Delayed ejaculation affects 4 % of sexually active men (Jannini et al. 2002).

CLASSIFICATION OF DIFFERENT FORMS

Retarded ejaculation can be drug-related or psychological (Hendry et al. 2000).

AETIOLOGY

Retarded ejaculation can be due to emotional suppression, an inability to relax, relationship difficulties, medications, societal and religious attitudes, and the use of alcohol and recreational drugs (1st Latin American Erectile Dysfunction Consensus Meeting, 2003c).

ROLE OF THE PELVIC FLOOR MUSCLES

During sexual activity, rhythmic contractions of the bulbocavernosus muscle along with the other pelvic floor muscles result in ejaculation (Gerstenberg et al. 1990). The external urethral sphincter and deep pelvic floor muscles relax rhythmically to allow the ejaculate to pass through the urethra. An inability to relax may compromise this process.

PREMATURE EJACULATION

Premature ejaculation is one of the commonest forms of sexual dysfunction (Rosen 2000). It is characterised by a lack of ejaculatory control and is associated with significant effects on sexual functioning and satisfaction (Rowland et al. 2004).

DEFINITION

Premature ejaculation has been defined as 'recurrent ejaculation that occurs with minimal stimulation and earlier than desired, before or soon after penetration, which causes bother or distress, and upon which the sufferer has little or no control' (World Health Organization 1992). It is also defined as 'the inability to delay ejaculation sufficiently to enjoy lovemaking. Persistent or recurrent occurrence of ejaculation with minimal sexual stimulation before, on, or shortly after penetration and before the person wishes it' (Hendry et al. 2000). Premature ejaculation is typically defined by three characteristics: short latency to ejaculation, lack of self-efficacy regarding the rapid ejaculation, and distress or dissatisfaction with the condition (Rowland 2003). Ejaculation may occur before or within 1 minute of the beginning of intercourse (Waldinger et al. 1998). It may occur in the absence of sufficient erection and the problem is not the result of prolonged abstinence from sexual activity.

CLASSIFICATION OF DIFFERENT FORMS

There are several different subtypes of biogenic and psychogenic premature ejaculation according to aetiological features (Metz & Pryor 2000). Physiological types of premature ejaculation are due to neurological constitution, acute physical illness, physical injury and pharmacological side-effect. Psychological types of premature ejaculation are due to psychological constitution, acute psychological distress, relationship distress and psychosexual skills deficit. Premature ejaculation may be labelled psychogenic when the physical cause is unknown.

PREVALENCE

The prevalence of premature ejaculation is 16.3% to 32.5% (Rowland et al. 2004). There is no evidence that ejaculation latency increases with age. In a stopwatch study of 110 men aged 18 to 65 years, 76% reported their ejaculation to be as rapid at their first sexual contacts with 23% reporting increasing rapidity and only 1% reporting a delay (Waldinger et al. 1998).

AETIOLOGY

The aetiology of premature ejaculation is unknown but psychological, behavioural and biogenic components are likely (Montague et al. 2004). There may be an organic basis for some forms of premature ejaculation. The causes can be congenital or acquired and/or psychological (1st Latin American Erectile Dysfunction Consensus Meeting, 2003c).

PATHOPHYSIOLOGY

Data suggests that men with premature ejaculation have hypersensitivity and hyperexcitability of the glans penis and the dorsal nerve (Xin et al. 1996, 1997).

ROLE OF PELVIC FLOOR MUSCLES

During sexual activity, rhythmic contractions of the bulbocavernosus muscle along with the other pelvic floor muscles result in ejaculation (Gerstenberg et al. 1990). Contraction of the pelvic floor muscles combined with intermittent relaxation of the external urinary sphincter and urogenital diaphragm allows ejaculation (Krane et al. 1989). The bladder neck sphincter under involuntary control remains closed. It is hypothesised that weak pelvic floor musculature affords little control to delay ejaculation and that the voluntary use of the pelvic floor muscles could delay ejaculation.

ASPERMIA

DEFINITION

Aspermia is defined as the absence of sperm at orgasm (Ralph & Wylie 2005).

AETIOLOGY

Aspermia is caused by an absent genital tract contraction (Ralph & Wylie 2005).

HAEMOSPERMIA

DEFINITION

Haemospermia is defined as blood in the semen (Ralph & Wylie 2005).

AETIOLOGY

In younger patients, under 40 years of age, haemospermia may result from infection in the urogenital tract. In older men, haemospermia in the absence of haematuria may result from cysts, calculi, polyps of the ejaculatory duct and seminal vesicles, and prostatic cancer (Ralph & Wylie 2005).

LOW-VOLUME EJACULATE

DEFINITION

Low-volume ejaculate is defined as an ejaculate volume of less than 1ml. Men with low-volume ejaculate wishing to father a child may be investigated for infertility.

AETIOLOGY

Low-volume or occasionally absent ejaculate may be caused by a deficiency of androgen from hypogonadal states or anti-androgen drugs. Other causes are urethral strictures, ejaculatory duct obstruction, congenital abnormalities of the seminal vesicles and vas deferens or neurological lesions from diabetes or surgery (Ralph & Wylie 2005).

PAINFUL EJACULATION

DEFINITION

Painful ejaculation is defined as pain during ejaculation (Ralph & Wylie 2005).

PREVALENCE

In an internet survey of 163 men with prostatitis, 69 % reported pain before or after ejaculation (Roehrborn et al. 2003).

AETIOLOGY

This uncommon problem may have psychological or organic causes. Organic causes may be prostatitis or, less commonly, ejaculatory duct obstruction, inflammation or stones (Ralph & Wylie 2005).

ANHEDONIA

DEFINITION

Anhedonia is defined as a total loss of feeling of pleasure during ejaculation (Ralph & Wylie 2005).

AETIOLOGY

Anhedonia may have psychological or organic causes.

SEXUAL PAIN

DEFINITION

Sexual pain is any pain which affects the ability to gain and maintain an erection and achieve orgasm and ejaculation.

AETIOLOGY

It may be due to urethritis, prostatitis, blockage to the seminal vesicles and/or hypertonic pelvic floor muscles (Chapter 7). Anal pain is from spasm of the external anal sphincter. Men with severe anal pain from anal fissures or haemorrhoids are unable to gain an erection owing to anal pain.

SUMMARY

Normal sexual function in men is dependent on satisfactory libido, erectile function, orgasm and ejaculation. Dysfunction may occur in any of these events. Sexual dysfunction embraces low libido, erectile dysfunction, premature ejaculation, retrograde ejaculation, retarded ejaculation, anorgasmia, anejaculation, aspermia, haemospermia, low-volume ejaculate, painful ejaculation, anhedonia and sexual pain.

15 Treatment of Male Sexual Dysfunction

Key points

- Male sexual dysfunction embraces low libido, erectile dysfunction and premature ejaculation.
- A range of treatment is available for erectile dysfunction.
- Couples are encouraged to choose the best option for their needs.
- All men should perform pelvic floor muscle exercises.
- Pelvic floor muscle exercises may be used in conjunction with other treatment.

INTRODUCTION

Male sexual dysfunction embraces low libido, erectile dysfunction and premature ejaculation. It can be treated in a number of ways.

LOW LIBIDO

Men with low libido who have hypogonadism can be treated with testosterone replacement therapy. Testosterone deficiency is confirmed by clinical features and biochemical tests. Gel from a sachet is applied daily to both shoulders, both arms or the abdomen. Testosterone patches placed daily on the skin can deliver testosterone to hypogonadal and ageing men. Dihydrotestosterone, synthesised from testosterone by 5-alpha-reductase activity, can also be used as a daily patch.

Contraindications for testosterone replacement therapy are those men with known or suspected prostate or breast cancer.

Undesirable effects include skin reactions, prostate changes and gynaecomastia. Female partners, especially pregnant women, should avoid contact with the gel application site and with gel-contaminated clothing.

ERECTILE DYSFUNCTION

A range of treatments are available for erectile dysfunction. Erectile dysfunction can be treated by using pelvic floor muscle exercises, oral medication, penile injections, intra-urethral and transglanular pharmacotherapy, vacuum devices and constriction rings, and surgery. Couples are advised to try out different methods before choosing the most suitable treatment for their needs.

ORAL MEDICATION

There are various forms of oral medication available for men with erectile dysfunction such as Viagra® (sildenafil citrate), Levitra® (vardenafil hydrochloride trihydrate), Cialis® (tadalafil), and Uprima® (apomorphine hydrochloride). All forms of oral therapy require men to be sexually stimulated or aroused. Sildenafil and vardenafil should be taken 30 to 60 minutes before sexual activity and the effectiveness lasts for about 4 hours. The effects of tadalafil last up to 36 hours and daily dosage may be used for a more natural response to sexual activity. Sildenafil, vardenafil and tadalafil are selective phosphodiesterase type 5 (PDE5) inhibitors which inhibit the breakdown of cGMP producing arterial vasodilation. The nitric oxide-cyclic guanosine-3'5'-monophosphate (NO/cGMP) system is important in producing the arterial dilation and venous occlusion necessary to attain and sustain an erection.

Oral medication may not be taken with nitrates such as glyceryl trinitrate which may have been prescribed for chest pains. Oral medication should not be taken more than once a day.

Side-effects include headaches, facial flushing, nasal congestion and dyspepsia.

Apomorphine can be given sublingually and acts centrally to promote an erection within 25 minutes. The side-effects of apomorphine are nausea in 15 % of men and more rarely vasa-vagal syndrome in 1 % of men.

PENILE INJECTIONS

The highly vasoactive substances papaverine, phentolamine and prostaglandin E1 (PGE1) are used in penile injections to produce penile rigidity. These drugs may be used separately or as a triple combination. The injection site is into either corpora cavernosum at the laterodorsal aspect of the proximal half of the penis.

Undesirable effects include burning during injection, prolonged erection, painful erection and penile fibrosis of erectile tissue. A prolonged erection lasting for more than 6 hours is considered to be an emergency and patients are strongly advised to consult a urologist urgently.

INTRA-URETHRAL PHARMACOTHERAPY

Intra-urethral and topical (transglanular) pharmacotherapy appear to play a role in the management of men with erectile dysfunction. The principal pharmacological agent has been MUSE® alprostadil the synthetic formulation of prostaglandin E1 (PGE1).

Undesirable effects are penile pain, headache, dizziness, symptomatic hypotension, minor urethral bleeding and testicular pain. Men are advised to wear a condom to prevent those partners who may be sensitive to alprostadil in the ejaculate from developing vaginitis.

VACUUM DEVICES

Negative pressure is applied to the penis from a vacuum pump cylinder pressed firmly against the pubis while vacuum is applied, then a constriction ring is placed at the base of the penis.

Undesirable effects include a cold penis, a pivoting base distal to the constriction band, pain during suction, pain and bruising at the ring site, pain at ejaculation and penile numbness.

LITERATURE REVIEW OF PHYSICAL THERAPY FOR ERECTILE DYSFUNCTION

The treatment of erectile dysfunction by physical therapists has been based on the evidence from a few trials. A literature review was undertaken to ascertain whether physical therapy had merit as a conservative treatment for erectile dysfunction.

LITERATURE SEARCH STRATEGY

A search of the following computerised databases from 1980 to 2005 was undertaken: Medline, AAMED (Allied and Alternative Medicine), CINAHL, EMBASE – Rehabilitation and Physical Medicine and The Cochrane Library Database. The keywords chosen were: *erectile dysfunction; impotence; conservative treatment; physical therapy; physiotherapy; pelvic floor exercises; biofeedback; electrical stimulation; electrotherapy.* A manual search was undertaken of identified manuscripts reporting on research studies gained from the references of this literature.

SELECTION CRITERIA

A study was included if the trial reported the results of physical therapy for men with erectile dysfunction and the outcome measures were reliable and relevant to the problem under investigation.

METHODOLOGICAL QUALITY

Methodological rigour was assessed from a hierarchy of evidence (Table 15.1).

EVIDENCE FOR THE EFFECT

Only two randomised controlled trials provided level II evidence that pelvic floor exercises cured or improved erectile function (Dorey et al. 2004a; Sommer et al. 2002). Five trials provided level III evidence (Claes & Baert 1993; Claes et al. 1995; Colpi et al. 1994; Mamberti-Dias & Bonierbale-Branchereau 1991; Van Kampen et al. 2003). Two trials solely used electrical stimulation and provided only level IV evidence (Derouet et al. 1998; Stief et al. 1996). (See Table 15.2.)

The trial by Sommer et al. (2002) used a large sample size of 124 men with venogenic erectile dysfunction. Men were randomised into three groups with one group receiving pelvic floor exercises, one group receiving Viagra® and one group receiving a placebo. At 3 months the pelvic floor exercise group improved more than the Viagra® group and significantly more than the placebo group. In the trial by Dorey et al. (2004a) 55 men were randomised into two groups with one group receiving pelvic floor exercises and one group receiving lifestyle changes. At 3 months the pelvic floor exercise group improved significantly compared to the control group. The control group were then given pelvic floor muscle exercises and they improved significantly when compared to their erectile function at baseline. Both groups continued home exercises for a further 3 months.

EFFECT SIZE

The two randomised controlled trials both showed significantly improved erectile function with pelvic floor muscle exercises. Sommer et al. (2002)

Table 15.1. Levels of evidence (Adapted from Sackett 1986)

I	Strong evidence from at least one systematic review of multiple well-designed randomised controlled trials
II	Strong evidence from at least one properly designed randomised controlled trial of appropriate size
III	Evidence from well-designed trials such as non-randomised trials, cohort studies, time series or matched case-control studies
IV	Evidence from well-designed non-experimental studies from more than one centre or research group
V	Opinions of respected authorities, based on the clinical evidence, descriptive studies or reports of expert committees

Table 15.2. Literature review of physical therapy for erectile dysfunction

Author/design	Subjects	Method	Outcomes
Mamberti-Dias & Bonierbale-Branchereau (1991) France *Sexologique* Not random No control **Level III evidence**	210 men with erectile dysfunction. Some with venous leakage. Some psychologic	PFMEs and electrical stimulation sacral and penile or perineal electrode 5–25 Hz then 50–400 Hz intermittent. Visual stimulation and penile temperature 15 treatments	**At 3 months** 111 (53 %) cured 44 (21 %) improved 55 (26 %) failed 67 % attained 4/10 to 8/10 ISMR (index of subjective mean rigidity) **Subjective outcome**
Claes & Baert (1993) Belgium *British Journal of Urology* Randomised No control	150 men with venogenic erectile dysfunction Age 23–64 Median age 48.7 Group 1 72 surgery Group 2 78 PFMEs	Group 1 Surgery deep dorsal vein Group 2 Patient education 5 weekly PFMEs Home exercises Digital anal assessment baseline, 4 and 12 months 40 mg papaverine + needle EMG ischiocavernosus muscle + maximum PFM contraction	**At 4 months** Group 1 44 (61 %) cured 17 (23.6 %) improved 11 (15.2 %) failed **At 4 months** Group 2 36 (46 %) cured 22 (28 %) improved 20 (25.6 %) failed **At 12 months** Group 1 30 (42 %) cured 23 (32 %) improved **At 12 months** Group 2 33 (42 %) cured 24 (31 %) improved 45 (58 %) refused surgery **Subjective and objective outcomes**
Level III evidence			

Table 15.2. *Continued*

Author/design	Subjects	Method	Outcomes
Colpi et al. (1994) Italy *Journal of Endocrinology Invest* Not random Controlled	59 men with venogenic erectile dysfunction Age 20–63 Mean age 39 Group 1 33 men PFMEs and biofeedback Group 2	30 of 59 deep dorsal vein surgery 30 of 59 psychological therapy No information which? No information on type of biofeedback	**At 11 months** Group 1 21 (63%) cured or improved Group 2 4 (15%) cured or improved 9 refused surgery
Level III evidence	26 men controls		**Subjective outcome**
Claes et al. (1995) Belgium *European Journal of Physical Medicine Rehabilitation* Not random No control	122 men with venogenic erectile dysfunction	Patient education PFMEs EMG or pressure biofeedback Electrical stimulation with anal or surface electrode, symmetrical biphasic low frequency 50-Hz pulse 100 μs 6 s stimulation 12 s rest maximum intensity	**At 4 months** 53 (43%) cured 37 (30%) improved 32 (26.2%) failed including 14 drop- outs **At 12 months** 44 (36%) cured 41 (33.6%) improved 37 (30.3%) failed including 14 drop- outs 65 (53.4%) refused surgery **Subjective outcome**
Level III evidence			

Study	Population	Intervention	Outcome
Stief et al. (1996) Germany *Urologe A* Not random Controlled **Level IV evidence**	22 men with erectile dysfunction who were vasoresponders	Transcutaneous electrical stimulation to smooth muscle corpus cavernosum. Low-frequency symmetrical trapezoidal 100–200µs 12mA alternating 10–20Hz and 20–35Hz 5s stimulation 2–5 days for 20 minutes	**At 5 days** 5 (23%) cured 3 (13.6%) responded to vaso-active drugs 14 (63%) failed **Subjective outcome**
Derouet et al. (1998) Germany *European Urology* Not random No Control **Level IV evidence**	48 men with erectile dysfunction	Transcutaneous electrical stimulation penile or perineal electrodes bipolar pulsed 85µs 30Hz 20–120mA 3s stimulation 6s rest 20 minutes daily for 3 months	**At 3 months** 5 (10.4%) cured 20 (41.6%) improved 23 (47%) failed including 10 drop-outs **Subjective improvement**
Sommer et al. (2002) Germany *European Urology Supplement* Randomised Controlled **Level II evidence**	124 men with venogenic erectile dysfunction Aged 21–72 Mean age 43.7 <u>Group 1</u> 40 men <u>Group 2</u> 36 men <u>Group 3</u> 28 men	<u>Group 1</u> 3 weekly PFMEs sessions <u>Group 2</u> Oral PDE5-inhibitor <u>Group 3</u> Placebo Outcome measures at baseline, 4 weeks and 3 months: KEED erectile dysfunction questionnaires, IIEF Q 3 and 4 and QoL At baseline and 3 months: caversonography	**At 3 months** <u>Group 1</u> 80% improved significantly 46% improved penile rigidity <u>Group 2</u> 74% improved <u>Group 3</u> 18% improved **Subjective and objective outcomes**

Table 15.2. *Continued*

Author/design	Subjects	Method	Outcomes
Van Kampen et al. (2003) Belgium *Physical Therapy* Not random No control **Level III evidence**	51 men with erectile dysfunction with mixed aetiology Age 25–64 Mean age 46	Patient education PFMEs in lying, sitting and standing. Anal pressure biofeedback. Electrical stimulation anal or surface electrode 50 Hz. 200 µs 6 s stimulation 12 s rest, once a week for 4 months. Home exercise, 90 contractions	**At 4 months** 24 (46 %) cured 12 (24 %) improved 15 (31 %) failed including drop-outs **Subjective outcome**
Dorey et al. (2004a) UK *British Journal of General Practice* Randomised Controlled **Level II evidence**	55 men with erectile dysfunction with mixed aetiology Age 22–78 Mean age 59 Intervention group 28 men PFMEs + lifestyle changes Control group 27 men lifestyle changes	Intervention group Patient education 5 weekly PFMEs and anal pressure biofeedback + home exercises + lifestyle changes Control group 5 weekly lifestyle changes. At 3 months control group given intervention. Outcome measures at 3 and 6 months: IIEF, ED-EQoL, anal manometry, blind assessment	**At 3 months** Erectile function domain of IIEF: intervention group significantly improved ($p = 0.001$) Control group ($p = 0.658$) Anal pressure: intervention group significantly improved ($p < 0.001$) **At 6 months** Blind assessment 22 (40 %) normal function including drop-outs 19 (34.5 %) improved including drop-outs 14 (25.5 %) failed including drop-outs **Subjective and objective outcomes**

Key: PFME = pelvic floor muscle exercises; EMG = electromyography; ISMR = Index of Subjective Mean Rigidity; PDE-5 = phosphodiesterase type 5; KEED = Kölner Erfassungsbogen für Erektile Dysfunktion; IIEF = International Index of Erectile Function; ED-EQoL = Erectile Dysfunction–Effect on Quality of Life.

found that the group of men who performed pelvic floor muscle exercises improved more than the group of men receiving oral PDE5-inhibitor (Viagra®) and significantly more than the group receiving a placebo (Figure 15.1). Dorey et al. (2004a) found at 3 months using the erectile function domain of the International Index of Erectile Function that the pelvic floor exercise group improved significantly ($p = 0.001$) compared with the control group ($p = 0.658$) (Figure 15.2). At 3 months, when the control group were given pelvic floor exercises they improved erectile function significantly ($p < 0.001$). This trial also found that the intervention group significantly improved anal pressure after 3 months pelvic floor exercises ($p < 0.001$) when compared to the control group.

CLINICAL SIGNIFICANCE

Both Sommer et al. (2002) and Dorey et al. (2004a) found that pelvic floor exercises improved erectile function clinically. Sommer et al. found that 46 % of men improved penile rigidity and Dorey et al. found that 40 % of men regained normal erectile function, and a further 34.5 % improved erectile function.

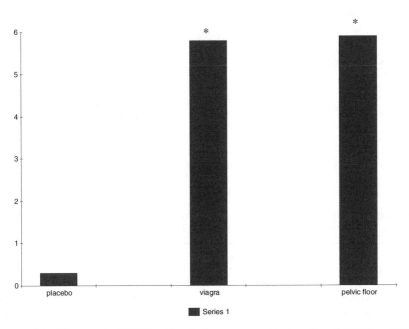

Figure 15.1. Changes in KEED at 3 months compared to baseline (KEED = Kölner Erfassungsbogen für Erektile Dysfunktion (Reproduced by permission of Sommer et al., 2002)

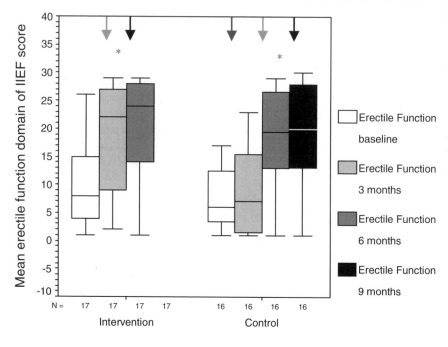

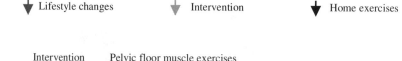

Figure 15.2. Mean erectile function domain of IIEF scores for both groups at each assessment (Reproduced by permission of John Wiley & Sons. *Source*: Dorey, 2004a)

METHODOLOGICAL QUALITY

The methodological quality was good in the two randomised controlled trials. The sample size was larger in the study by Sommer et al. (2002). Sommer et al. (2002) used men with proven venogenic erectile dysfunction. Dorey et al. (2004a) used men with a wide range of aetiology. Both used validated subjective outcome measures and, unlike the other trials, both used objective outcome measures.

The results from the uncontrolled or non-randomised trials should be interpreted with caution because of the poor methodology. Only one of these trials used randomisation, five of the trials lacked controls and seven provided only subjective outcomes. Unfortunately, the lack of control groups in these trials impinged on the validity of evidence provided. The lack of randomisation is an important methodological limitation which fundamentally limited any definitive interpretation and translation of the findings from these trials.

TYPE OF INTERVENTION

There was only one trial which used pelvic floor exercises alone (Sommer et al. 2002). This trial provided good results without biofeedback and questions the need for biofeedback. Two trials included biofeedback as the only other modality (Colpi et al. 1994; Dorey et al. 2004a), whilst two combined pelvic floor muscle exercises with biofeedback and electrical stimulation (Claes et al. 1995; Van Kampen et al. 2003). It is impossible to determine which modality has caused the effect when three modalities are used.

The amount of pelvic floor exercise varied. Colpi et al. (1994) expected men to perform daily home exercises for 30 minutes a day for 9 months as a realistic alternative to surgery. Dorey et al. (2004a) instructed men to perform 18 strong contractions a day with emphasis on functional work. No trial mentioned a long-term follow-up or advised a maintenance programme for life, although Claes and Baert (1993), and Claes et al. (1995) followed up subjects for 12 months with encouraging results.

Two trials used electrical stimulation alone. Derouet et al. (1998) found electrical stimulation to the ischiocavernosus muscle produced only a 10.4 % cure rate whilst Stief et al. (1996) in a controlled trial explored transcutaneous electrical stimulation to the smooth muscle of the penile corpus cavernosum and obtained a 23 % cure rate. Whatever effect was achieved, both cure rates were low compared to the pelvic floor muscle exercise trials.

FREQUENCY AND DURATION OF TRAINING

The amount of treatment varied from between 5 and 20 treatment sessions, although some papers did not provide this information. Sommer et al. (2002) treated men in three weekly pelvic floor muscle exercise sessions and monitored the men at 4 weeks and 3 months. Dorey et al. (2004a) treated men in five weekly pelvic floor exercise sessions and monitored the men at 3 months and at 6 months. In both studies men performed home exercises.

SHORT- AND LONG-TERM EFFECTS

From the available data, it appears that patients were assessed initially, and then at between 3 and 12 months. The exception to this was the trial by Stief et al. (1996) where outcomes were assessed after 5 days.

Both Sommer et al. (2002) and Dorey et al. (2004a) used the subjective validated International Index of Erectile Function which is used extensively for trials using oral medication for erectile dysfunction. Sommer et al. (2002) used the validated Kölner Erfassungsbogen für Erektile Dysfunktion (KEED). Dorey et al. (2004a) used an assessor who was blinded to the subject group to report trial outcomes. Mamberti-Dias and Bonierbale-Branchereau (1991) used an index of subjective mean rigidity (ISMR) and reported an increase from 4 out of 10 to 8 out of 10 mean ISMR.

Most outcomes used patient reported 'cure', 'improved' or 'failure'. 'Cure' was defined as an erection suitable for satisfactory sexual performance with vaginal penetration in all studies. 'Improvement', however, was defined in a number of ways from 'a significant increase of erection quality and performance' (Colpi et al. 1994) to 'partial response for those patients who reported some increase in quality (duration or rigidity) of erections but not sufficient for sexual intercourse' (Claes et al. 1995).

Three trials used objective outcome measurements. Claes and Baert (1993) injected 40 mg papaverine to achieve penile rigidity and tested with needle EMG whilst contracting the ischiocavernosus muscle maximally. Sommer et al. (2002) used Rigiscan as an objective measurement of penile rigidity and Dorey et al. (2004a) used anal manometric biofeedback readings.

Sommer et al. (2002) used a quality of life instrument and Dorey et al. (2004a) used the validated Erectile Dysfunction–Effect on Quality of Life (ED-EQoL) (MacDonagh et al. 2002). Dorey et al. (2004a) found there was poor correlation of the IIEF with the ED-EQoL in the intervention group but significant correlation in the control group. This finding showed that erectile dysfunction may have impacted on men in different ways and demonstrated a clear reason for the clinical usefulness of a quality of life questionnaire.

The short-term effects were good in all the trials of pelvic floor exercises for erectile dysfunction. The two randomised controlled trials have provided good results at 3 months (Sommer et al. 2002; Dorey et al. 2004a) and 6 months (Dorey et al. 2004a). The results were good at 12 months in the trial by Claes and Baert (1993).

PSYCHOSEXUAL ISSUES

All the trials used a sample of heterosexual men. No study mentioned any cultural factors. The perceptions of sexual activity vary from one man to another and impact on the expectations and the subjective measurement of sexual performance. Not all men wish to practise penetrative sex. There were no studies which identified and addressed the difficulties and needs of homosexual men who practise anal intercourse.

RECOMMENDATIONS BASED ON EVIDENCE

Pelvic floor exercises should be the first-line treatment for erectile dysfunction (Figure 15.3). They may be performed in conjunction with other treatment for erectile dysfunction, such as oral therapy, vacuum devices, intra-cavernosus injections, intra-urethral medication, constriction bands and counselling.

CONSERVATIVE MANAGEMENT FOR THE PREVENTION OF ERECTILE DYSFUNCTION

There were no publications using preventative conservative treatment. However, if the pelvic floor musculature is poor, and pelvic floor muscle exercises can relieve erectile dysfunction, then it seems reasonable to suppose that preventative muscle strengthening may help to prevent erectile dysfunction.

CONCLUSIONS

There is grade II level evidence that pelvic floor muscle exercises seem to have merit as a treatment for erectile dysfunction. There is grade III evidence of

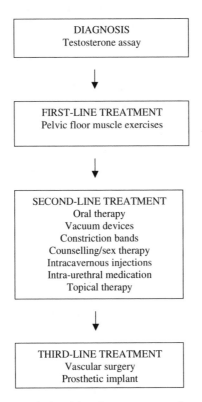

Figure 15.3. Suggested algorithm for treatment of erectile dysfunction

similar results. For those patients who appear to have been cured or improved with pelvic floor muscle exercises, it may be prudent to continue these simple exercises for life and possibly avoid a return of erectile dysfunction. However, long-term compliance may be a problem. Following initial pelvic floor training, it may be possible to maintain muscle performance with a minimal exercise programme.

There was no strong evidence that electrical stimulation was effective in the treatment of erectile dysfunction.

No studies demonstrating preventative conservative treatment were found for these men.

A multi-centred randomised controlled trial with larger sample numbers is needed to explore the use of pelvic floor exercises as a first-line treatment for men with erectile dysfunction. Similar trials are also needed to ascertain the role of pelvic floor exercises as prophylaxis for erectile dysfunction.

PREMATURE EJACULATION

A literature review was undertaken to ascertain whether pelvic floor muscle exercises may have merit as a treatment for premature ejaculation.

LITERATURE SEARCH STRATEGY

A search of the following computerised databases from 1980 to 2005 was undertaken: Medline, AAMED (Allied and Alternative Medicine), CINAHL, EMBASE – Rehabilitation and Physical Medicine and The Cochrane Library Database. The keywords chosen were: *premature ejaculation; conservative treatment; physical therapy; physiotherapy; pelvic floor exercises; biofeedback; electrical stimulation; electrotherapy.* A manual search was also undertaken.

SELECTION CRITERIA

A study was included if it reported the results of physical therapy for men with premature ejaculation.

METHODOLOGICAL QUALITY

Methodological rigour was assessed from a hierarchy of evidence (Table 15.1).

RESULTS

Two non-randomised uncontrolled trials were found providing level III evidence (LaPera & Nicastro 1996; Claes & van Poppel 2005) (Table 15.3).

Table 15.3. Literature review of physical therapy for premature ejaculation

Author/design	Subjects	Method	Outcomes
La Pera & Nicastro (1996) Italy *Journal of Sex and Marital Therapy* Non-randomised No control **Level IV evidence**	18 men with premature ejaculation Aged 20–52 Mean age 34	Pelvic floor exercises Pressure biofeedback Electrical stimulation Anal probe 50 Hz 3 times a week for 20 sessions	**At 7 weeks** 11 (61 %) cured 7 (39 %) no improvement **Subjective and objective outcomes**
Claes & van Poppel (2005) Belgium *Journal of Sexual Medicine* Non-randomised No control **Level IV evidence**	29 men with premature ejaculation Age not disclosed	Pelvic floor exercises Electrical stimulation Parameters not given Ejaculatory latency time Method of measurement not given	**After treatment** 19 (65.5 %) improved 10 (34.5 %) failed to improve **At 12 months** Most of the 19 who improved still showed a positive response **Subjective outcomes**

METHODOLOGY

La Pera and Nicastro (1996) used pelvic floor muscle exercises, pressure bio-feedback and electrical stimulation in a non-randomised and uncontrolled trial of 18 patients with a mean age of 34 years (range 20–52 years) to treat premature ejaculation. Results showed that 11 patients (61 %) were cured and reported improved pelvic floor muscle control whilst 7 (39 %) showed no improvement. Unfortunately, the biofeedback readings were not given. This non-randomised, uncontrolled study has shown that there may be merit in strengthening the pelvic floor muscles to control the ejaculatory reflex and prevent premature ejaculation. In this trial 18 patients were recruited, including 15 men who had experienced premature ejaculation for over 5 years.

In a non-randomised uncontrolled trial, Claes and van Poppel (2005) investigated the action of pelvic floor exercises and electrical stimulation on 29 men with premature ejaculation. After treatment, they found that 19 men (65.5 %) showed improvement which was verified by their partner. At 12 months, most of the men who had improved still showed a positive result.

METHODOLOGICAL QUALITY

The methodology used in these two trials lacked randomisation and a control group and included a small sample size to provide only weak evidence.

However, results from these trials indicated that this subject is worth further exploration.

RECOMMENDATIONS

Randomised controlled trials need to be undertaken of pelvic floor muscle exercises for premature ejaculation before any conclusions can be made.

CONCLUSIONS

A range of treatment is available for men with erectile dysfunction. Grade II evidence has shown that pelvic floor muscle exercises are effective for erectile dysfunction and should be the first-line treatment option. They may be used in conjunction with other forms of therapy.

Weak evidence indicates that the use of pelvic floor muscle exercises for premature ejaculation is worth further exploration.

16 Setting up a Continence Service

Key points

- The continence service should comprise the director of continence services, continence nurse specialists, specialist continence physiotherapists, designated medical and surgical specialists, and investigation and treatment facilities.
- The director may be a continence specialist physiotherapist or a continence nurse specialist with the necessary qualifications and clinical experience.

INTRODUCTION

An integrated continence service should provide a good-quality service accessible to all men without undue waiting time. Patients should be able to move seamlessly from one professional to another as appropriate.

INTEGRATED CONTINENCE SERVICES

Continence services for a specific population should be organised as integrated continence services (Department of Health 2000). Various professionals at different levels may be employed by different bodies but should be integrated into a locally provided continence service. The continence service should comprise the director of continence services, continence nurse specialists, specialist continence physiotherapists, designated medical and surgical specialists, and investigation and treatment facilities.

Each Health Authority should have access to integrated continence services, managed by a director of continence services who would usually be a continence nurse specialist or specialist continence physiotherapist responsible for:

- overseeing and co-ordinating the development and implementation of common policies, procedures and protocols;
- developing and maintaining care pathways to and from primary care and specialist services;
- ensuring users and carers are involved in all aspects of the service;

- ensuring services are made available to all residents in the area served;
- working closely with other services such as social services, education services and psychological services;
- ensuring services are made available to all patients in hospital who require them;
- co-ordinating educational activities for continence specialists, primary health care teams and others involved in the delivery of health and social care;
- organising service-wide review, audit and research activities particularly to ensure national targets are met;
- promoting awareness of continence (Department of Health 2000).

The Association for Continence Advice has produced a file and CD-ROM entitled 'Steps to Success' dealing with all issues concerned with setting up a continence service (ACA 2004).

INTERDISCIPLINARY COLLABORATION

For best practice, physiotherapists, continence advisors, urology nurses, urologists and GPs need to collaborate and provide an interdisciplinary service for male patients with lower urinary tract symptoms.

In 1998 a consensus forum of key UK representatives from nurses and physiotherapists working in the specialised field of continence compiled a bipartite statement identifying the collaboration between the two professions (Interprofessional Collaboration in Continence Care 1998). A need to establish a working party to define core competencies and develop mutual education needs was identified. This collaboration was seen as an important breakthrough in the mutual understanding and roles of the two professions and served as a basis for future networking for the benefit of the patient.

For interdisciplinary working to be successful it is essential that all disciplines are involved in free discussion and careful audit of the service (Haslam 1996). Collaborative exchanges on patient care must be the model for the future. A continence service should include referral from any member of the interdisciplinary team and include self-referral. In conjunction with the wishes of the patient access should be available to any of the team who are specialised in male continence care. The network of team members is shown in Table 16.1.

The shared-care model provides a good example of how medical specialists and allied health professionals can work together to provide comprehensive health care of a high standard.

(Halloran 1991)

Table 16.1. Interdisciplinary team involved in a continence service

Continence advisor
Continence nurse specialist
Health visitor
Specialist continence physiotherapist
Occupational therapist
Dietician
Social worker
Urologist
Geriatrician
Neurologist
General practitioner
Consultant in rehabilitation
Psychiatrist
Clinical psychologist
Coloproctologist
Gastroenterologist
Supplies staff
Voluntary bodies
Users and carers

DIRECTOR OF CONTINENCE SERVICES

The director of continence services should be a continence nurse specialist or a specialist continence physiotherapist who has had considerable experience in the speciality of continence, who has good management experience and who is able to provide training for members of staff at primary care and secondary care levels.

QUALIFICATIONS

There is a Masters level physiotherapy specific continence course at the University of Bradford. The award of Postgraduate Certificate: Continence for Physiotherapists requires the successful completion of two 20-credit core modules and a further 20-credit module from a choice available within the School of Health Studies. The award forms part of the MSc Rehabilitation Studies programme. Further studies can be undertaken towards the full award of MSc Rehabilitation Studies. The core modules consist of theoretical and practical components delivered in residential blocks and appropriate clinical settings. The work-based learning component comprises 150 hours of clinical practice.

The University of the West of England runs an MSc Advanced Practice programme. Nurses or physiotherapists may choose to study continence-related issues for each of the modules. Students may study for a Post-Graduate

Certificate or take further modules to be awarded a Post-Graduate Diploma or be awarded an MSc Advanced Practice with further study and a dissertation.

Some universities are encouraging nurses and physiotherapists to study continence in an Independent Study Programme leading to an MSc award.

MEMBERSHIP OF SPECIALIST GROUPS

The specialist continence physiotherapist or continence nurse specialist would be expected to be a member of one or more of the following groups, which provide lectures and courses on continence. All these groups provide benefits to their members such as a directory of specialists, a journal or newsletter, shared knowledge from courses and conferences, networking, details of current research literature, continence promotions, posters and patient leaflets.

Association for Continence Advice (ACA)

A group for nurses and physiotherapists working in the specialist area of continence.

Association of Chartered Physiotherapists in Women's Health (ACPWH)

A clinical interest group of the Chartered Society of Physiotherapy for physiotherapists working in women's health.

Chartered Physiotherapists Promoting Continence (CPPC)

A clinical interest group of the Chartered Society of Physiotherapy for physiotherapists treating male and female continence patients.

United Kingdom Continence Society (UKCS)

A group which includes doctors, scientists, nurses, physiotherapists and technicians from the UK, who are interested in presenting, sharing and hearing the recent research findings.

International Continence Society (ICS)

An international group of doctors, scientists, nurses, physiotherapists and technicians who share outcomes from current research.

CONTINUING PROFESSIONAL DEVELOPMENT

The specialist continence physiotherapist or continence nurse specialist would be expected to attend study days and conferences in order to show evidence of continuing professional development or lifelong learning. The following conferences provide current continence information and evidence on which to base practice:

ACA Conference
ACPWH Conference
CPPC Study Days
Male and Female Continence Study Days
UKCS Annual Scientific Meeting
ICS Annual Meeting

BUDGET

The following items need to be considered when budgeting for a continence service:

Staff salaries
Staff training
Investigative equipment
Biofeedback equipment
Electrical stimulation equipment
Anal pressure probes, anal electrodes and surface electrodes
Medical sundries, such as condoms, non-latex gloves and gel
Pad service
Continence appliances
Advertising costs
Patient information leaflet costs
Additional costs for stationery, photocopying etc

BUSINESS PLAN

The following considerations should form part of a business plan:

Justification for providing a quality service
The internal customers (inpatients, outpatients, home visits, residential homes)
The external customers (consultants, GPs, carers and other professionals)
Budget
Audit
Evaluation of services

MARKETING

In order to market the continence service, other professionals and interested parties should be targeted:

Hospital managers
Consultants and GPs
Other nurses, well-man screenings, prostate clinics
Other physiotherapists
The public

The continence service can be advertised by:

Leaflets
Posters
Open days
Lectures to the public
Local paper
Local radio
Local cinema
Local TV

CONTACTS FOR SPECIALIST GROUPS

CPPC Chartered Physiotherapists Promoting Continence

c/o The Chartered Society of Physiotherapy
14 Bedford Row
London WC1R 4ED
Telephone: 020 7306 6666

ACA Association for Continence Advice

Meeting Makers Ltd
Jordan Hill Campus
76 South Brae Drive
Glasgow G13 1PP
Scotland
Telephone: 0141 434 1500
Email: carol@meetingmakers.co.uk

ACPWH Association of Chartered Physiotherapists in Women's Health

c/o The Chartered Society of Physiotherapy
14 Bedford Row
London WC1R 4ED
Telephone: 020 7306 6666

Royal College of Nursing Continence Care Forum

20 Cavendish Street
London W1M 0AB
Telephone: 020 7409 3333

United Kingdom Continence Society (UKCS)

Myra Glass Secretary ICS (UK) or
Ian Ramsay Honorary Secretary/Treasurer ICS (UK)
Dept. of Gynaecology
Southern General Hospital
1345 Govan Road
Glasgow G51 4TF
Website: www.icsuk.org.uk

ICS International Continence Society

ICS Office
Southmead Hospital
Bristol BS10 5NB
Telephone: 0117 950 3510
Website: www.icsoffice.org

SUPPLIERS

Model of the male pelvic floor to show patients

Educational and Scientific Products Ltd
A2 Dominion Way
Rustington
West Sussex BN16 3HQ
Telephone: 01903 773340

ANUFORM™ rectal probe

NEEN Mobilis Healthcare Group
100 Shaw Road
Oldham OL1 4AY
Telephone: 0161 627 4401

HELPLINES FOR MEN IN THE UK

The Prostate Cancer Charity

3 Angel Walk
Hammersmith

London W6 9HX
Telephone: 0845 300 8383
Website: www.prostate-cancer.org.uk

Prostate Help Association

Langworth
Lincoln LN3 5DF
Website: www.pha.u-net.com

The British Prostate Support Association

1 Walcote House
Sandy Lane
Royal Leamington Spa
Warwickshire CV32 6QS
Website: www.bps-assoc.org.uk

The Continence Foundation

307 Hatton Square
16 Baldwins Gardens
London EC1N 7RJ
Telephone: 0845 345 0165
Website: www.continence-foundation.org.uk

Incontact (National Action on Incontinence)

United House
North Road
London N7 9DP
Telephone: 020 7700 7035

British Association of Sex and Relationship Therapy

PO Box 13686
London SW20 9ZH

Relate

Relate Central Office
Herbert Gray College
Little Church Street
Rugby
Warwickshire CV21 3AP

Sexual Dysfunction Association

Windmill Place Business Centre
2–4 Windmill Lane
Southall
Middlesex UB2 4NJ
Telephone: 0870 774 3571
Website: www.sda.uk.net

NHS smoking helpline

Telephone: 0800 169 0169

BOOKS AND VIDEOS FOR PROFESSIONALS

Incontinence
  Volume 1: *Basic and Evaluation*
  Volume 2: *Management*
Editors: P. Abrams, L. Cardozo, S. Khoury, A. Wein
Health Publications Ltd, 2005
Distributor: Editions 21
76 rue de la Pompe
75016 Paris
France
Email: editions21@wanadoo.fr

Pelvic Floor Exercises for Erectile Dysfunction
Author: G. Dorey
John Wiley & Sons Ltd
The Atrium
Southern Gate
Chichester
West Sussex PO19 8SQ
Telephone: 01243 779777

Professional assessment video or DVD
Subjective assessment of post radical prostatectomy patient
Dorey, G., Foreman, K.
Dr K. Foreman
Studio 222, The Citadel
Bath Road
Chippenham
Wiltshire SN15 2AB, UK

Email: kevin.foreman@uwe.ac.uk
Website: www.winhealth.co.uk

Professional assessment video or DVD
Demonstration of digital anal assessment of male pelvic floor muscles
Website: www.winhealth.co.uk

BOOKS FOR PATIENTS

Use it or lose it! (second edition)
Self-help book for men with urinary leakage or erectile dysfunction
Author: Dr Grace Dorey
NEEN Mobilis Healthcare Group
100 Shaw Road
Oldham OL1 4AY
Telephone: 0161 925 3180
Website: www.mobilishealthcare.com

Living and Loving after Prostate Surgery
Author: Professor Grace Dorey
Old Hill Farm
Portmore
Barnstaple
Devon EX32 0HR
Telephone: 01271 321721
Email: grace.dorey@virgin.net

Prostate Cancer: A Comprehensive Guide for Patients
Jane Smith, Raj Persad, Kieran Jefferson
TFM Publishing
Website: www.amazon.com

Prevent it!
A guide for men and women with leakage from the back passage
Author: Dr Grace Dorey
NEEN Mobilis Healthcare Group
100 Shaw Road
Oldham OL1 4AY
Telephone: 0161 925 3180
Website: www.mobilishealthcare.com

Clench it or Drench it! **(second edition)**
A self-help guide for ladies who lunch, laugh and leak
Using your pelvic floor muscles to overcome urinary leakage

Professor Grace Dorey
Old Hill Farm
Portmore
Barnstaple
Devon EX32 0HR
Telephone: 01271 321721
Email: grace.dorey@virgin.net

Stronger and longer!
Improving erections with pelvic floor exercises
Professor Grace Dorey
Old Hill Farm
Portmore
Barnstaple
Devon EX32 0HR
Telephone: 01271 321721
Email: grace.dorey@virgin.net

VIDEO FOR PATIENTS

Men's Health Video
Self-help video for men with erectile dysfunction and post-micturition dribble
Video of patient performing pelvic floor muscle exercises
Foreman, K., Dorey, G.
Dr K. Foreman
Studio 222, The Citadel
Bath Road
Chippenham
Wiltshire SN15 2AB, UK
Email: kevin.foreman@uwe.ac.uk
Website: www.winhealth.co.uk

SUMMARY

The continence service should comprise the director of continence services, continence nurse specialists, specialist continence physiotherapists, designated medical and surgical specialists, and investigation and treatment facilities. The director may be a continence specialist physiotherapist or a continence nurse specialist with the necessary qualifications and clinical experience.

Appendix: Male Continence Assessment Form

Patient details		
Name		
Address		
Telephone numbers		
DoB / Age		
Occupation		
Physical hobbies / activities		
Source of referral		
Surgical history		
TURP	Date	Outcome
Radical prostatectomy	Date	Outcome
Urethral stricture	Date	Outcome
Other surgery	Date	Outcome
Radiotherapy		
Problems		
Main problem		
Length of time for main problem		
Mild	Moderate	Severe
Improvement or deterioration to date		
Other problems		
Limitation to activities		

QoL due to urinary problem
Bothersome rating   0   1   2   3   4   5   6   7   8   9   10
Symptoms
Stress urinary incontinence
Urgency
Urge urinary incontinence
Provoking factors
Aware of leakage
Daytime frequency
Nocturia
Nocturnal enuresis
Poor sensation of micturition
Slow stream
Intermittent stream
Hesitancy
Straining
Terminal dribble
Post-micturition dribble
Continuous urinary incontinence
Need to double void
Does bladder feel empty after voiding
Dysuria
Haematuria, dark or smoky urine
Pain: suprapubic, genital, perineal, testis, penis (mark on body chart)
Amount of leakage
Few drops   Spurt   Large leakage

No. of pads per day	Size of pads	Small	Medium	Large
No. of pads at night	Size of pads	Small	Medium	Large

Sheath system

Intermittent self-catheterisation

Indwelling catheter	Size	Number of days used

Frequency of leakage

Daily	>1 / week	<1 / week	>1 / month	<1 / month

Time of day leakage occurs

Leakage aggravators Coughing Sneezing Walking Moving Running water Caffeine Alcohol Medication Other:

Urine stop test (not to be used as an exercise)

Stop	Slow down	Unable to stop

Bowel activity

Constipation

Straining to defaecate

Number of times defaecates per week

Stool consistency	Liquid	Soft	Firm

Faecal urgency

Faecal leakage

Control of flatus

Laxatives

Diet

Medical history

Prostatitis	Acute	Chronic	No. of episodes
Cystitis	Acute	Chronic	No. of episodes

Latex allergy

Metal implants

Heart problems
Blood pressure
Smoking
Respiratory problems
Other problems
Medication
Anticholinergic medication Tolterodine (Detrusitol) Oxybutynin (Ditropan)
Alpha-blockers (relax bladder neck) Tamulosin, Alfuzosin, Doxazosin (Cardura)
5-alpha reductase inhibitors (reduces prostate size) Finasteride (Proscar)
Anti-androgen drug treatment Goserelin, Leuprorelin
Cholinergic agonists enhance detrusor contractions Carbachol and Bethanechol
Other medications
Effect of medication
Side-effects of medication
Neurological problems
Diabetes   MS   Parkinson's   Stroke   Other:
Lumbar or cervical spine problems with neurological deficit
Previous treatment
Physiotherapy treatment   Outcome
Body Mass Index
Height   metres
Weight   kilograms
BMI (weight in kilograms divided by height in metres squared) >30 = obese
Sexual problems
Difficulty gaining erection
Difficulty maintaining erection

Wakes with an erection	Times out of 7
Premature ejaculation	
Functional factors	
Position used for urination	
Mobility and dexterity	
Environmental factors	
Patient support system	
Motivation	
Ability to incorporate therapy into lifestyle	
Investigations	
Urinalysis of mid-stream urine	
Prostate specific antigen	
Uroflow	
Post-void residual	
Ultrasound scan	
Urodynamics	
Flexible cystoscopy	
24-hour pad test	
Bladder diary	
Daytime frequency	
Nocturia	
Maximum voided volume	
Minimum voided volume	
Total fluid intake	
Amount of caffeine intake	
Amount of alcohol intake	

Total urinary output				
Time of going to bed				
Amount voided at night				
Frequency of leakage				
Number of pads per day				
Informed consent				
Chaperone present	Yes		No	
Abdominal palpation				
Full bladder after voided urine				
Abnormal pelvic mass				
Abdominal pain				
Perineal and genital examination in supine lying with knees bent				
Congenital abnormality				
Skin condition	Penis	Perineum	Scrotum	Anus
Evidence of infection				
Ability to tighten anus				
Penile retraction and testicular lift				
Leakage on coughing				
Ability to prevent leakage on coughing				
Dermatomes				
S2 lateral buttocks and thigh, posterior calf and plantar heel			Right	Left
S3 upper two-thirds of medial thigh			Right	Left
S4 penis and perineal area			Right	Left
S5 anal sphincter			Right	Left
Myotomes				
External anal sphincter S2, 3			Right	Left

Levator ani Ischiococcygeus Bulbocavernosus S2, 3, 4	Right	Left

Bulbocavernosus reflex test

Gentle pressure on glans penis during a digital anal examination elicits anal sphincter contraction unless neurological impairment

DIGITAL ANAL EXAMINATION

Anterior

O

Posterior

Anal sphincter strength   0 1 2 3 4 5 6
Anal sphincter endurance
Puborectalis strength   0 1 2 3 4 5 6
Puborectalis endurance
Ability to perform fast contraction

Problems
1
2
3
4

Patient identified goals of treatment
1
2
3
4

Treatment
1
2
3
4

Advice
1
2
3
4

Plan
1
2
3
4

Questions for next time
1
2
3
4

Name of physiotherapist _____

Signature _____

Date _____

Glossary

ACA Association for Continence Advice

ACPWH Association of Chartered Physiotherapists in Women's Health

anejaculation absence of ejaculation during orgasm

anhedonia loss of pleasure during ejaculation

anodyspareunia painful receptive anal intercourse

anorgasmia inability to achieve orgasm

antimuscarinic medication blocks muscarinic receptors in detrusor muscle

aspermia absence of sperm at orgasm

AVP arginine vasopressin

biofeedback monitors muscle activity to encourage greater effort

bladder diary records voided volumes, incontinence episodes and fluid intake

BMI body mass index (over 30 is obese)

BOO bladder outlet obstruction

BPE benign prostatic enlargement

BPH benign prostatic hyperplasia

cardiac arrhythmia irregular heartbeat

clam ileoplasty bladder augmentation using portion of ileum

cm H$_2$O centimetres of water

CPPC Chartered Physiotherapists Promoting Continence

CranioSacral Therapy gentle manual technique to realign spinal cord and nerve roots

Credé's manoeuvre leaning forward with pressure on the abdomen whilst straining to void

cycloplegia blurred vision

cystometry tests relationship between volume and pressure in bladder during filling and voiding

cystourethroscopy endoscopic investigation of the bladder and urethra

DAE digital anal examination

deep dorsal vein incision ligature of penile vein to reduce venous outflow from the penis

defaecation elimination of waste products from the body

detrusor/sphincter dyssynergia spasm of the internal urethral sphincter whilst the bladder is contracting

dihydrotestosterone synthesis of testosterone

dysuria pain on passing urine

ED-EQoL Erectile Dysfunction Effect on Quality of Life questionnaire

electrical stimulation   stimulation to achieve a muscle contraction

EMG   electromyogram; monitoring muscle activity by electronic means using skin, anal or needle electrode

epispadias   congenital abnormality of urethra meatus opening dorsally

epistaxis   nosebleed

erectile dysfunction   inability to achieve or maintain an erection sufficient for satisfactory performance

faeces   waste products of digestion

flatus   wind from the back passage

F/V chart   frequency/volume chart

GP   general practitioner

gynaecomastia   development of breasts in a man

haemospermia   blood in semen

hypospadias   congenital abnormality of urethra meatus opening ventrally

Hz   hertz; unit of frequency of electrical current

iatrogenic   (trauma) caused by surgery or medication

ICS   International Continence Society

ICS*QoL*   International Continence Society quality of life questionnaire

ICS*sex*   International Continence Society sex questionnaire

idiopathic   having no known cause

IIEF   International Index of Erectile Function questionnaire

IIQ-7   International Incontinence Questionnaire – 7

I-PSS   International Prostate Symptom Score

ISC   intermittent self-catheterisation

ISIR   International Society of Impotence Research

ISMR   index of subjective mean rigidity (measure of penile rigidity by the patient)

isometric contraction   static contraction of muscle with same length

isotonic contraction   dynamic contraction of muscle with same tone

IVP   intravenous pyelogram

KEED   Kölner Erfassungsbogen für Erektile Dysfunktion questionnaire

KUB   kidneys, ureters and bladder

libido   sexual urge

LUTS   lower urinary tract symptoms

mg bd   milligrams twice a day

mg qds   milligrams four times a day

mg td   milligrams three times a day

ml   millilitre

mmHg   millimetres of mercury

ms   milliseconds

MS   multiple sclerosis

MSU   mid-stream urine

myofascial release   gentle manual techniques for muscles and fascial coverings

natriuresis excretion of sodium ions

ng/ml nanograms per millilitre

NI nocturia index

NIH National Institutes of Health

NPI nocturnal polyuria index

NUV nocturnal urine volume

orchidectomy surgical removal of the testes

PFMs pelvic floor muscles

PFMEs pelvic floor muscle exercises (contractions of all the pelvic floor muscles)

PFMT pelvic floor muscle training

pH potential of hydrogen; a measure of the acidity or alkalinity of a solution

PMD post-micturition dribble

PNF proprioceptive neuromuscular facilitation

PNV predicted number of nightly voids

premature ejaculation ejaculation with minimal stimulation earlier than desired

PSA prostate-specific antigen

Q_{max} maximum urinary flow rate

QoL quality of life

RCT randomised controlled trial

retarded ejaculation delay in reaching climax

retrograde ejaculation backward passage of semen into bladder

sacral neuromodulation electrical stimulation of peripheral nerves from implanted stimulator

saw palmetto *Serenoa repens* plant extract for benign prostatic hyperplasia

storage symptoms symptoms experienced during storage phase of bladder

tachycardia increased heartbeat

TURP transurethral resection of prostate

urodynamics study of pressure, volume and flow relationships in the lower urinary tract

μV microvolt

valsalva manoeuvre bearing down as if defaecating

voiding symptoms symptoms experienced during the voiding phase of the bladder

WHO World Health Organisation

xanthines natural diuretics such as caffeine and theobromine

References

1st Latin American Erectile Dysfunction Consensus Meeting (2003a) Androgen deficiency in the aging male *International Journal of Impotence Research* 15(Suppl. 7):S12–S15

1st Latin American Erectile Dysfunction Consensus Meeting (2003b) Anatomy and Physiology of erection: pathophysiology of erectile dysfunction *International Journal of Impotence Research* 15(Suppl. 7):S5–S8

1st Latin American Erectile Dysfunction Consensus Meeting (2003c) Psychogenic erectile dysfunction and ejaculation disorders *International Journal of Impotence Research* 15(Suppl. 7):S16–S21

Abrams, P (1995) Managing lower urinary tract symptoms in older men *British Medical Journal* 310:1113–1117

Abrams PA, Blaivas JG, Stanton SL, Andersen JT (1998) Standardization of the lower urinary tract function *Neurourology and Urodynamics* 7:403

Abrams P, Cardozo L, Fall M, Griffiths D, Rosier P, Ulmsten U, van Kerrebroeck P, Victor A, Wein A (2002a) The standardisation of terminology of lower urinary tract function: report from the Standardisation Sub-committee of the International Continence Society *Neurourology and Urodynamics* 21:167–178

Abrams P, Cardozo L, Khoury S, Wein A (2002b) *Incontinence* 2nd International Consultation, Published by Plymbridge Distribution Ltd, Plymouth, England

ACA (2004) *Steps to Success* SUI/173, Association for Continence Advice, London

ACA Survey (Association for Continence Advice Survey of Patients National Care Audit) (2000) Association for Continence Advice, London

Addison R (1997) Cranberry juice: the story so far *Journal of the Association of Chartered Physiotherapists in Women's Health* 80:21–22

Albaugh J, Lewis JH (1999) Insights into the management of erectile dysfunction: Part I *Urologic Nursing* 19(4):241–247

Andersen KV, Bovim G (1997) Impotence and nerve entrapment in long distance amateur cyclists *Acta Neurologica Scandinavica* 95(4):233–240

Anderson RU, Wise D, Meadows M (1999) Myofascial release therapy for category III prostatitis. www.prostatitis.org/myofascialrel.html

Andersson KE, Wein AJ (2005) Pharmacology of the lower urinary tract – basis for current and future treatments of lower urinary incontinence *Pharmacology Review* (in press)

Andrew J, Nathan PW, Spanos NC (1964) Cerebral cortex and micturition. *Proceedings of the Royal Society of Medicine* 58:533

Arvedson J (1930) *Medical Gymnastics and Massage in General Practice* 3rd edn. Dobbie ML (ed.) Churchill, London, 276–287

Ashton-Miller JA, DeLancey JOL (1996) The Knack: use of precisely-timed pelvic muscle contraction can reduce leakage in SUI *Neurourology and Urodynamics* 15(4):392–393

Avorn J, Monane M, Gurwitz JH, Glynn RJ, Choodnovskiy I, Lipsitz LA (1994) Reduction of bacteriuria and pyuria after ingestion of cranberry juice *Journal of American Medical Association* 271:751–754

Aytac IA, McKinlay JB, Krane RJ (1999) The likely worldwide increase in erectile dysfunction between 1995 and 2025 and some possible policy consequences *British Journal of Urology International* 84:50–56

Bales GT, Gerber GS, Minor TX, Mhoon DA, McFarland JM, Kim HL, Brendler CB (2000) Effect of preoperative biofeedback/pelvic floor training on continence in men undergoing radical prostatectomy *Urology* 56(4):627–630

Baniel J, Israilov S, Shmueli J, Segenreich E, Livne PM (2000) Sexual function in 131 patients with benign prostatic hyperplasia before prostatectomy *European Urology* 38(1):53–58

Barnas JL, Pierpaoli S, Ladd P, Valenzuela R, Aviv N, Parker M, Bedford Waters W, Flanigan C, Mulhall JP (2004) The prevalence and nature of orgasmic dysfunction after radical prostatectomy *British Journal of Urology International* 94:603–605

Beachy EH (1981) Bacterial adherence: adhesion receptor inter-actions mediating the attachment of bacteria to mucosal surfaces *Journal of Infectious Diseases* 143:325–345

Beckett SD et al. (1973) Blood pressures and penile muscle activity in the stallion during coitus *American Journal of Physiology* 225:1072–1075

Benet AE, Melman A (1995) The epidemiology of erectile dysfunction *Urologic Clinics of North America* 22:699–709

Bennett JK, Foote JE, Green BG, Killorin EW, Martin SH (1997) Effectiveness of biofeedback/electrostimulation in treatment of post-prostatectomy urinary incontinence. Abstract Presentation, Urodynamics Society, New Orleans, April 1997

Bensignor MF, Labat JJ, Robert R, Ducrot P (1996) Diagnostic and therapeutic pudendal nerve blocks for patients with perineal non-malignant pain. Abstract, 8th World Congress on Pain, 56

Berger AP, Deibl M, Leonhartsberger N et al. (2005) Vascular damage as a risk factor for benign prostatic hyperplasia and erectile dysfunction *British Journal of Urology International* 96:1073–1078

Berger Y (1995) Urodynamic studies. In: Fitzpatrick JM, Krane RJ (eds) *The Bladder* Churchill Livingstone, London, 47–70

Berghmans LCM, Hendriks HJM, Bø K, Hay-Smith EJ, de Bie RA, van Waalwijk van Doorn ESC (1998) Conservative treatment of stress urinary incontinence in women: a systematic review of randomized clinical trials *British Journal of Urology* 82:181–191

Bernstein IT (1997) The pelvic floor muscles: muscle thickness in healthy and urinary-incontinent women measured by perineal ultrasonography with reference to the effect of pelvic floor training. Estrogen Receptor Studies *Neurourology and Urodynamics* 16:237–275

Blaivas JG, Appell RA, Fanti, JA, Leach G, McGuire EJ, Resnick NM, Raz S, Wein AJ (1997) Definition and classification of urinary incontinence: recommendations of the Urodynamic Society *Neurourology and Urodynamics* 16:149–151

Bodel PT, Cotran R, Kass EH (1959) Cranberry juice and antibacterial action of hippuric acid *Journal of Laboratory and Clinical Medicine* 54(6):881–888

Bortolotti A, Parazzini F, Colli E, Landoni M (1997) The epidemiology of erectile dysfunction and its risk factors *International Journal of Andrology* 20(6): 323–334

Branch LG, Walker LA, Wetle TT, DuBeau CE, Resnick NM (1994) Urinary incontinence knowledge among community-dwelling people 65 years of age and older *Journal of the American Geriatric Society* 42(12):1257–1262

Britton JP, Dowell AC, Whelan P (1990) Prevalence of urinary symptoms in men aged over 60 *British Journal of Urology* 66:175–176

Brock GB, Lue TF (1993) Drug-induced male sexual dysfunction: an update *Drug Safety* 8(6):414–426

Brocklehurst JC (1993) Urinary incontinence in the community – analysis of a MORI poll *British Medical Journal* 306:832–834

Bruce JM (1899) *The Principles of Treatment and Their Applications in Practical Medicine* Young J Pentand, London, 215–224

Burgio K (2002) Influence of behaviour modification on overactive bladder *Urology* 60(5):72–76

Burgio KL, Stutzman RE, Engel BT (1989) Behavioral training for post-prostatectomy urinary incontinence *The Journal of Urology* 141:303–306

Caldamone AA (1994) Embryology. In: Sant GR (ed.) *Pathophysiologic Principles of Urology* Blackwell Scientific Publications: London, 1–29

Cancer Research UK (2005) Prostate cancer. www.cancerresearchuk.org

Cash JE (1957) *Physiotherapy in Some Surgical Conditions* Faber & Faber, London, 78–79

Castleden CM, Duffin HM, Gulati RS (1986) Double blind study of imipramine and placebo for incontinence due to bladder instability *Age Ageing* 15:299–303

Chadwick AJ, Mann WN (1987) Hippocrates: Airs waters and places. In: Chadwick AJ, Mann WN (eds) *Hippocratic Writings* Penguin, London, 47–64

Chamberlain J, Melia J, Moss S, Brown J (1997) Report prepared for the health technology assessment panel of the NHS executive on the diagnosis, management, treatment and costs of prostate cancer in England and Wales *British Journal of Urology* 79(3):1–32

Chapple CR, Parkhouse H, Gardner G, Milroy EJG (1990) Double-blind, placebo controlled cross over study of flavoxate in the treatment of idiopathic detrusor instability *British Journal of Urology* 66:491–494

Chartered Society of Physiotherapy (2005) Prescribing rights for physiotherapists – an update. Chartered Society of Physiotherapy, London, PA 58

Chaudry AA, Booth CM, Holmes A, Al-Dabbagh MA (1997) Are urodynamics essential for the management of 'prostatism'? Two patient group studies *British Journal of Urology* 79(Suppl. 4):18

Christensen H, Fuglsang-Frederiksen A (1998) Quantitative surface EMG during sustained and intermittent submaximal contractions *Electroencephalography in Clinical Neurophysiology* 70(3):239–247

Christiansen J, Rasmussen Ø, Lindorff-Larsen K (1998) Dynamic graciloplasty for severe anal incontinence *British Journal of Surgery* 85:88–91

Christiansen J, Rasmussen Ø, Lindorff-Larsen K (1999) Long-term results of artificial anal sphincter implantation for severe anal incontinence *Annals of Surgery* 230:45–48

Chute CG, Panser LA, Girman CJ, Oesterling JE, Guess HA, Jacobson, SJ (1993) The prevalence of prostatism: a population-based survey of urinary symptoms *Journal of Urology* 150:85–89

Claes H, Baert L (1993) Pelvic floor exercise versus surgery in the treatment of impotence *British Journal of Urology* 71:52–57

Claes H, Bijnens B, Baert L (1996) The hemodynamic influence of the ischiocavernosus muscles on erectile function *Journal of Urology* 156:986–990

Claes H, Van Kampen M, Lysens R, Baert L (1995) Pelvic floor exercises in the treatment of impotence *European Journal of Physical Medicine Rehabilitation* 5:135–140

Claes HI, Van Poppel H (2005) Pelvic floor exercise in the treatment of premature ejaculation *The Journal of Sexual Medicine* 2(Suppl. 1):9

Claesson B, Siosteen A, Nordholm L (1999) PNF in physiotherapy of today and tomorrow – a survey of Swedish physiotherapists *Nordisk Fysioterapi* 3(1):3–12

Colpi GM, Negri L, Nappi RE, Chinea B (1999) Perineal floor efficiency in sexually potent and impotent men *International Journal of Impotence Research* 11(3):153–157

Colpi GM, Negri L, Scroppo FI, Grugnetti C (1994) Perineal floor rehabilitation: a new treatment for venogenic impotence *Journal of Endocrinology Invest* 17:34

Consensus Statement (1997) First International Conference for the Prevention of Incontinence. Danesfield House, UK, June 25–27. The Continence Foundation, London

Craggs MD, Chaffer NJ, Mundy AR (1991) A preliminary report on a new hydraulic sphincter for controlling urinary incontinence *Journal of Medical Engineering and Technology* 15(2):58–62

Davidson PJT, van den Ouden D, Schroeder FH (1996) Radical prostatectomy: prospective assessment of mortality and morbidity *European Urology* 29:168–173

De Castro R, Ricci G, Gentili A, Miniero R, Di Lorenzo F, Pigna A, Masi M (1999) Latex allergy in patients who had undergone multiple surgical procedures for urinary bladder exstrophy: preliminary data *British Journal of Urology International* 83(Suppl. 3):96(Abstract)

DeLancey J (1994) Functional anatomy of the pelvic floor and urinary continence mechanism. In: Schüssler B, Laycock J, Norton P, Stanton S (eds) *Pelvic Floor Re-education, Principles and Practice* Springer-Verlag, London, 9–21

Denmeade SR, Lin XS, Isaacs JT (1996) Role of programmed (apoptotic) cell death during the progression and therapy for prostate cancer *Prostate* 28:251–265

Denning J (1996) Male urinary continence. In: Norton C (ed.) *Nursing for Continence* Beaconsfield Publishers Ltd, Beaconsfield, UK, 153–169

Department of Health (2000) *Good Practice in Continence Services* Department of Health, London

De Ridder D, Chandiramini V, Dasgupta P, Van Poppel H, Baert L, Fowler C (1997) Intravesical capsaicin as a treatment for refractory detrusor hyperreflexia *Journal of Urology* 158(6):2087–2092

Derouet H, Nolden W, Jost WH, Osterhage J, Eckert RE, Ziegler M (1998) Treatment of erectile dysfunction by an external ischiocavernosus muscle stimulator *European Urology* 34(4):355–359

Dinubile NA (1991) Strength training *Clinical Sports Medicine* 10(1):33–62

Dixon J, Gosling J (1994) Histomorphology of pelvic floor muscle. In: Shussler B, Laycock J, Norton P, Stanton S (eds) *Pelvic Floor Re-education. Principles and Practice* Springer-Verlag, London, 28–33

Djavan B, Madersbacher S, Klinger HC, Ghawidel K, Basharkhah A, Hruby S, Seitz C, Marberger M (1999) Outcome analysis of minimally invasive treatments for benign prostatic hyperplasia *Techniques in Urology* 5(1):12–20

Djurhuus JC, Matthiesen TB, Rittig S (1999) Similarities and dissimilarities between nocturnal enuresis in childhood and nocturia in adults *British Journal of Urology International* 84(Suppl. 1):9–12

Dolman M (2003) Normal and abnormal bladder function. In: Getliffe K, Dolman M (eds) *Promoting Continence: A Clinical and Research Resource* Baillière Tindall, London

Donnellan SM, Duncan HJ, MacGregor RJ, Russell JM (1997) Prospective assessment of incontinence after radical retropubic prostatectomy: objective and subjective analysis *Urology* 49(2):225–230

Donovan JL, Abrams P, Peters TJ (1996) The ICS-'BPH' Study: the psychometric validity and reliability of the ICS*male* questionnaire *British Journal of Urology* 77:554–562

Donovan JL, Kay HE, Peters TJ et al. (1997) Using ICS*Qol* to measure the impact of lower urinary tract symptoms on quality of life: evidence from the ICS-'BPH' study. *British Journal of Urology* 80:712–721

Dorey G (1998) Physiotherapy for male continence problems *Physiotherapy* 85(11):556–563

Dorey G (2000) Physiotherapy for the relief of male lower urinary tract symptoms: a Delphi study *Physiotherapy* 86(8):413–426

Dorey G (2001a) Is smoking a cause of erectile dysfunction? A review of the literature *British Journal of Nursing* 10(7):455–465

Dorey G (2001b) *Conservative treatment of Male Urinary Incontinence and Erectile Dysfunction.* Whurr Publishers, London, 1–170

Dorey G (2004a) *Pelvic Floor Muscle Exercises for Erectile Dysfunction.* Whurr Publishers, London, 1–129

Dorey G (2004b) *Prevent it!* Book for men and women with faecal leakage. NEEN Mobilis Healthcare Group, Oldham, 1–28

Dorey G (2005) *Living and Loving after Prostate Surgery.* Dorey G (ed.) Barnstaple, Devon, 1–26

Dorey G, Speakman M, Feneley R, Dunn C, Swinkels A, Ewings P (2004a) Randomised controlled trial of pelvic floor muscle exercises and manometric biofeedback for erectile dysfunction *British Journal of General Practice* 54(508): 819–825

Dorey G, Speakman M, Feneley R, Dunn C, Swinkels A, Ewings P (2004b) Randomised controlled trial of pelvic floor muscle exercises and manometric biofeedback for post-micturition dribble *Urologic Nursing* 24(6):490–512

Dorey G, Swinkels A (2003) Test retest reliability of anal pressure measurements in men with erectile dysfunction *Urologic Nursing* 23(3):204–212

Dunsmuir WD, Emberton M, Neal DE, on behalf of the steering group of the National Prostatectomy Audit (1996) There is no sexual satisfaction following TURP *British Journal of Urology* 77:161A

Ebbell B (1937) *The Papyrus Ebers. The Greatest Egyptian Medical Document* Levin & Munksgaard, Copenhagen, 1–111

Eberhart NM (1920) *A Working Manual of High Frequency Currents* 6th edn. New Medicine Publishing Co., Chicago, 252–253

Edmonds SF (1991) Preparing for the return home; discharge information following prostatectomy *Professional Nurse* October:29–30

Elbadawi A (1995) Pathology and pathophysiology of the detrusor in incontinence *Urologic Clinics of North America* 22:499–512

Elbadawi A, Schenk EA (1974) A new theory of the innervation of bladder musculature. Part 4. Innervation of the vesicourethral junction and external urethral sphincter *Journal of Urology* 111:613

Elder DD, Stephenson TP (1980) An assessment of the Frewen Regime in the treatment of detrusor dysfunction in females *British Journal of Urology* 52:467–471

Elliman, Sons & Co. (1903) Rubbing Eases Pain. *The REP Book*. 2nd edn. Elliman, Sons and Co, Slough, 199–203

Emberton M, Meredith P, Wood C, Ellis BW, Kinton D, Neal DE (1997) An interactive CD-ROM multi-media patient information package for men with lower urinary symptoms *Royal College of Surgeons of England*, London, UK

Emberton M, Neal DE, Black N, Fordham M, Harrison M, McBrien MP, Williams RE, McPherson K, Devlin HB (1996) The effect of prostatectomy on symptom severity and quality of life *British Journal of Urology* 77(2):233–247

Engel AF, Kamm MA, Bartram CI (1995) Unwanted anal penetration as a physical cause of faecal incontinence *European Journal of Gastroenterology and Hepatology* 7(1):65–67

Fabra M, Porst H (1999) Bulbocavernosus-reflex latencies and pudendal nerve SSEP compared to penile vascular testing in 669 patients with erectile failure and sexual dysfunction *International Journal of Impotence Research* 11(3):167–175

Fall M, Lindstrom S (1991) Electrical stimulation: a physiological approach to the treatment of urinary incontinence *Urologic Clinics of North America* 18(2):393–407

Fantel JA, Wyman JF, Harkins SW (1990) Bladder training in the community – dwelling incontinent population *Journal of American Geriatrics Society* 38:282–288

Feldman HA, Goldstein I, Hatzichristou DG et al. (1994) Impotence and its medical and psychological correlates: results of the Massachusetts Male Ageing Study *Journal of Urology* 151:54–61

Fellers CR, Redmon BC, Parrott RN (1933) Effect of cranberries on urinary acidity and blood alkali reserve *Journal of Nutrition* 6:455

Feneley RCL (1986) Post Micturition Dribbling. In: Mandelstam D (ed.) *Incontinence and its Management* Croom Helm, London

Fisher C, Gross J, Zuch J (1965) Cycle of penile erections synchronous with dreaming (REM) sleep *Archives of General Psychiatry* 12:29–45

FitzGerald MP, Kotarinos R (2003) Rehabilitation of the short pelvic floor: II: Treatment of the patient with the short pelvic floor *International Urogynecology Journal* 14:269–275

Fonda D (1999) Nocturia: a disease or normal ageing? *British Journal of Urology International* 84(Suppl. 1):13–15

Ford H (1992) Feeling off colour: colour of urine and faeces indicate disease *Nursing Times* 89(5):64–68

Franke JJ, Gilbert WB, Grier J et al. (2000) Early post prostatectomy pelvic floor biofeedback *Journal of Urology* 163:191–193

Frankel SJ, Donovan JL, Peters TJ, Abrams P, Dabhoiwala NF, Osawa D, Tong Long Lin A (1998) Sexual dysfunction in men with lower urinary tract symptoms *Journal of Clinical Epidemiology* 51:677–685

Frewen W (1979) Role of bladder training in the treatment of the unstable bladder in the female *Urologic Clinics of North America* 6:273

Friedman DM (2003) The demon rod. In: Friedman DM (ed.) *A Mind of Its Own: A Cultural History of the Penis* Robert Hale, London, 1–42

Gadsby G (1998) Electroanalgesia: historical and contemporary developments. PhD thesis. http://freespace.virgin.net/joseph.gadsby/page11.htm

Gardiner D (1959) *The Principles of Exercise Therapy* 2nd edn. Bell, London, 150–151

Gardiner D (1964) *Physiotherapy Target for Careers* 1st edn. Hale, London, 78–81

Garraway WM, Collins GN, Lee RJ (1991) High prevalence of benign prostatic hypertrophy in the community *Lancet* 338:469–471

Garrison FH (1917) *History of Medicine* 2nd edn. WB Saunders Co, London, 736

Garry RC, Roberts TDM, Todd JK (1959) Reflexes involving the external urethral sphincter in the cat *Journal of Physiology* 149:635–665

Gee WF, Ansell JS, Bonica JJ (1990) Pelvic and perineal pain of urologic origin. In: Bonica JJ (ed.) *The Management of Pain* Vol. 2. Lea & Febiger, Philadelphia, 1368–1394

Geirsson G, Fall M (1997) Maximal functional electrical stimulation in routine practice *Neurourology and Urodynamics* 16:559–565

Gerstenberg TC, Levin RJ, Wagner G (1990) Erection and ejaculation in man. Assessment of the electromyographic activity of the bulbocavernosus and ischiocavernosus muscles *British Journal of Urology* 65:395–402

Gordon H, Logue M (1985) Perineal muscle function after childbirth *The Lancet* 1–2, 8441–8450:123–125

Gosling JA, Dixon JS, Critchley HOD, Thompson SA (1981) A comparative study of the human external sphincter and periurethral levator ani muscle *British Journal of Urology* 53:35–41

Gray H (1858) *Anatomy: Descriptive and Surgical* Parker & Son, London

Gray H (1909) *Anatomy: Descriptive and Surgical* Pickering Pick T (ed.) Parker & Son, London

Gray M (1992) *Genitourinary Disorders* Mosby's Clinical Nursing Series Mosby Year-Book Inc., St Louis, MO

Gray ML (1996) Genitourinary embryology, anatomy and physiology. In: Karlowicz K (ed.) *Urologic Nursing: Principles and Practice* 1st edn. Saunders, Philadelphia

Gray ML (1998) Neurophysiology of the bladder. 4th National Multi-speciality Nursing Conference, Orlando, FL

Griffiths DJ, Holstege G, Dalm E, de Wall H (1990) Control and coordination of bladder and urethral function in the brainstem of the cat *Neurourology and Urodynamics* 9:63–92

Guyton AC (1986) *Textbook of Medical Physiology* W.B. Saunders, Philadelphia, 1013–1014

Habib NA, Luck RJ (1983) Results of transurethral resection of the benign prostate. *British Journal of Urology* 70:218–219

Haidinger G, Temml C, Schatzl G, Brossner C, Roehlich M, Schmidbauer CP, Madersbacher S (2000) Risk Factors for Lower Urinary Tract Symptoms in Elderly Men *European Urology* 37:413–420

Halaska M, Dorschner W, Frank M (1994) Treatment of urgency and incontinence in elderly patients with propiverine hydrochloride *Neurourology and Urodynamics* 13:428–430

Halloran J (1991) The shared-care model *Medical Journal of Australia* 155:614

Harrison SCW, Abrams P (1994) Bladder function. In: Sant GR (ed.) *Pathophysiologic Principles of Urology* Blackwell Scientific Publications, New York

Haslam EJ (1999) Evaluation of pelvic floor muscle assessment, digital, manometric and surface electromyography in females. MPhil thesis, University of Manchester, UK

Haslam J (1996) Working together *Nursing Times* 92(15):68

Haslam J (1998) Physiotherapy EMG/biofeedback. The 2nd International Association for Continence Advice Conference, Edinburgh (Abstract)

Haslam J, Jeyaseelan S, Oldham JA, Roe BH (1998) Inter-tester reliability for digital assessment of the pelvic floor. 5th Annual Meeting, International Continence Society(UK) Cambridge, UK, 2nd–3rd April (Abstract)

Hayden, LJ (1993) Chronic testicular pain *Australian Family Physician* 22:1357–1365

Hendry WF (1999) Causes and treatment of ejaculatory disorders. In: Carson CC, Kirby RS, Goldstein I (eds) *Textbook of Erectile Dysfunction* Isis Medical Media, Oxford, 569–581

Hendry WF, Althof SE, Benson GS, Haensel SM, Hull EM, Kihara K, Opsomer RJ (2000) Male orgasmic and ejaculatory disorders. In: Jardin A, Wagner G, Khoury S, Giuliano F, Padma-Nathan H, Rosen R (eds) *Erectile Dysfunction* Health Publication Ltd, Plymbridge Distributors Ltd, Plymouth, UK, 479–506

Heruti R, Shochat T, Tekes-Manova D, Ashkenazi I, Justo D (2004) Prevalence of erectile dysfunction among young adults: results of a large-scale survey *Journal of Sexual Medicine* 1:284–291

Hirakawa S, Hassouna M, Deleon R, Elhilali M (1993) The role of combined pelvic floor stimulation and biofeedback in post-prostatectomy urinary incontinence (Abstract 87) *Journal of Urology* 149:235A

Holland JM, Feldman JL, Gilbert HC (1994) Phantom orchialgia *Journal of Urology* 152:2291–2293

Holley RL, Varner RE, Kerns DJ, Mestecky PJ (1995) Long-term failure of pelvic floor musculature exercises in treatment of genuine stress incontinence *South Medical Journal* 88(5):547–549

Hunsballe J, Ritting S, Pedersen E, Olesen O, Djurhuus J (1997) Single dose imipramine reduces nocturia *Journal of Urology* 158:830–836

Hunter DJ, Berra-Unamuno A, Martin-Gordo A (1996) Prevalence of urinary symptoms and other urological conditions in Spanish men 50 years old or older *Journal of Urology* 155(6):1965–1970

Hunter KF, Moore KN, Cody DJ, Glazener CMA (2004) Conservative management for postprostatectomy urinary incontinence (Cochrane Review). In: *The Cochrane Library* Issue 3. John Wiley, Chichester, UK

Interprofessional Collaboration in Continence Care (ICCC) (1998) *Nurses and Physiotherapists Working in Continence Care* Report of a Consensus Meeting held at the King's Fund London. Association for Continence Advice, London

Intili H, Nier D (1998) Self-esteem and depression in men who present with erectile dysfunction. *Urologic Nursing* 18(3):185–187

Jackson J, Emerson L, Johnston B, Wilson J, Morales A (1996) Biofeedback: a non-invasive treatment for incontinence after radical prostatectomy *Urologic Nursing* 16(2):50–54

Jannini EA, Simonelli C, Lenzi A (2002) Sexological approach to ejaculatory dysfunction *International Journal of Andrology* 25:317–323

Jezernik S, Craggs M, Grill WM, Creasey G, Rijkhoff NJ (2002) Electrical stimulation for the treatment of bladder dysfunction: current status and future possibilities *Neurological Research* 24(5):413–430

Jones R (1994) Neuromuscular adaptability: therapeutic implications *Journal of the Association of Physiotherapists in Obstetrics and Gynaecology* 75:12–17

Joseph AC, Chang MK (2000) Comparison of behavior therapy methods for urinary incontinence following prostate surgery: a pilot study *Urologic Nursing* 21:203

Kaplan SA, Santarosa RP, D'Alisera PM, Fay BJ, Ikeguchi EF, Hendricks J, Klein L, Te AE (1997) Pseudodyssynergia (contraction of the external sphincter during voiding) misdiagnosed as chronic nonbacterial prostatitis and the role of biofeedback as a therapeutic option *Journal of Urology* 157:2234–2237

Karacan I, Aslan C, Hirshkowitz M (1983) Erectile mechanisms in man *Science* 220:1080

Kawanishi Y, Yamaguchi K, Kishimoto T, Nakatsuji H, Kojima K, Yamamoto A, Numata A (2000) Simple evaluation of ischiocavernous muscle *International Journal of Impotence Research* 12(Suppl. 2):13

Keane D, O'Sullivan S (2000) Urinary incontinence: anatomy, physiology and pathophysiology. In: Cardozo L (ed.) *Clinical Obstetrics and Gynaecology* Baillière Tindall, Harcourt Health Sciences, London

Kegel A (1948) Progressive resistance exercise in the functional restoration of the perineal muscles *American Journal of Obstetrics and Gynecology* 56:238–248

Kegel AH (1956) Early genital relaxation *Obstetrics and Gynecology* 8(5):545–550

Kinney AB, Blount M (1979) Effect of cranberry juice on urinary pH *Nursing Research* 28(5):287–290

Kirby R, Carson C, Goldstein I (1999) Anatomy, physiology and pathophysiology. In: Kirby R (ed.) *Erectile Dysfunction: A Clinical Guide* Isis Medical Media, Oxford, 11–28

Kirby R, Fitzpatrick J, Kirby M, Fitzpatrick A (eds) (1994) *Shared Care for Prostatic Diseases* Isis Medical Media, Oxford, 16

Knight S (2005) Chronic pelvic pain in men and women: Is the pelvic floor a common link? *Journal of the Association of Chartered Physiotherapists in Women's Health* 96:16–27

Knight SJ, Laycock J (1994) The role of biofeedback in pelvic floor re-education *Physiotherapy* 80:145–148

Knight SJ, Laycock J (1998) Evaluation of neuromuscular electrical stimulation in the treatment of genuine stress incontinence *Physiotherapy* 84(2):61–71

Knott M, Voss DE (1968) In: Knott M, Voss DE (eds) *Proprioceptive Neuromuscular Facilitation* 2nd edn. Harper & Row, New York, 188–189

Koeman M, Van Driel MF, Weijmar Schultz WCM, Mensink HJA (1996) Orgasm after radical prostatectomy *British Journal of Urology* 77:861–864

Kortmann BBM, Sonke GS, D'Ancona FCH, Floratos DL, Debruyne FMJ, de la Rosette JJMCH (1999) The tolerability of urodynamic studies and flexible cysto-urethroscopy used in the assessment of men with lower urinary tract symptoms. *British Journal of Urology* 84:449–453

Krane RJ, Goldstein I, Saenz De Tejada I (1989) Medical progress: impotence *New England Journal of Medicine* 321:1648–1659

Krauss DJ, Lilien OM (1981) Transcutaneous electrical nerve stimulation for stress incontinence *Journal of Urology* 125(6):790–793

Krieger JN, Nyberg L, Nickel JC (1999) Consensus definition and classification of prostatitis *Journal of American Medical Association* 282(3):236–237

La Pera G, Nicastro A (1996) A new treatment for premature ejaculation: the rehabilitation of the pelvic floor *Journal of Sex and Marital Therapy* 22(1):22–26

Lavoisier P, Courtois F, Barres D, Blanchard M (1986) Correlation between intracavernous pressure and contraction of the ischiocavernosus muscle in man *Journal of Urology* 136:936–939

Lawrence WT, MacDonagh RP (1988) Treatment of urethral stricture disease by internal urethrotomy followed by intermittent 'low friction' self-catheterisation *Journal of the Royal Society of Medicine* 81(3):136–139

Leaver RB (1996) Cranberry juice *Professional Nurse* 11(8):525–526

Le Lievre S (1999) Care of the incontinent client's skin *Journal of Community Nursing* 14(2):26–32

Levin RM, Wein AJ (1995) Neurophysiology and Neuropharmacology. In: Fitzpatrick JM, Krane RJ (eds) *The Bladder* Churchill Livingstone, London, 47–70

Lewis RW, Mills TM (1999) Risk factors for impotence. In: Carson CC, Kirby RS, Goldstein I (eds) *Textbook of Erectile Dysfunction* Isis Medical Media, Oxford, 141–148

Light JK, Rapoll E, Wheeler TM (1997) The striated urethral sphincter: muscle fibre types and distribution in the prostatic capsule *British Journal of Urology* 79:539–542

Lizza EF, Rosen RC (1999) Definition and classification of erectile dysfunction: report of the Nomenclature Committee of the International Society of Impotence Research *International Journal of Impotence Research* 11(3):141–143

LoPiccolo J (1986) Diagnosis and treatment of male sexual dysfunction *Journal of Marital Therapy* 11:215–232

MacDonagh R, Ewings P, Porter T (2002) The effect of erectile dysfunction on Quality of Life: psychometric testing of a new Quality of Life measure for patients with erectile dysfunction *Journal of Urology* 167:212–217

Mahady IW, Begg BM (1981) Long term symptomatic and cystometric care of the urge incontinence syndrome using a technique of bladder re-education *British Journal of Obstetrics and Gynecology* 88:1038–1043

Mahony DT, Laferte RO, Blais DJ (1977) Integral storage and voiding reflexes *Neurology* 9(1):95–106

Malmsten UGH, Milsom I, Molander U, Norlen LJ (1997) Urinary incontinence and lower urinary tract symptoms: an epidemiological study of men aged 45 to 99 years. *Journal of Urology* 158:1733–1737

Malone-Lee JG (2000) The efficacy, tolerability and safety profile of tolterodine in the treatment of overactive/unstable bladder *Reviews in Contemporary Pharmacotherapy* 11:29–42

Mamberti-Dias A, Bonierbale-Branchereau M (1991) Therapy for dysfunctioning erections: four years later, how do things stand? *Sexologique* 1:24–25

Mamberti-Dias A, Vasavada SP, Bourcier AP (1999) *Pelvic Floor Dysfunction: Investigations and Conservative Treatment* Casa Editrice Scientifica Internazionale, Rome, 303–310

Mathewson-Chapman M (1997) Pelvic muscle exercise/biofeedback for urinary incontinence after prostatectomy: an education program *Journal of Cancer Education* 12(4):218–223

McArdle WD, Catch FI, Catch VL (1991) *Exercise Physiology* 2nd edn. Lea & Febinger, Philadelphia, 1–12

McGuire EJ, O'Connell HE (1995) The bladder and spinal cord injury. In: Fitzpatrick JM, Krane RJ (eds) *The Bladder* Churchill Livingstone, New York, 213–227

Metz ME, Pryor JL (2000) Premature ejaculation: a psychophysiological approach for assessment and management *Journal of Sex and Marital Therapy* 26(4):293–320

Middlekoop HAM, Smilde-van den Doel DA, Neven AK, Kamphuisen HAC, Springer CP (1996) Subjective sleep characteristics of 1,485 males and females aged 50–93: effect of sex and age and factors related to self-evaluated quality of sleep *Journal of Geronology* 51A:108–115

Millard RJ (1989) After-dribble. In: Millard RJ (ed.) *Bladder Control – A Simple Self-help Guide* Williams & Wilkins, NSW, Australia, 89–90

Millard RJ, Oldenburg BF (1983) The symptomatic, urodynamic and psychodynamic results of bladder re-education programs *Journal of Urology* 130:715–719

Miller J, Ashton-Miller JA, DeLancey JOL (1996) The Knack: use of precisely-timed pelvic muscle contraction can reduce leakage in SUI *Neurourology and Urodynamics* 15(4):392–393

Millin T, Read CD (1948) Stress incontinence of urine in the female *Post Graduate Medical Journal* 3–10

Milne JS, Williamson J, Maule MM (1972) Urinary symptoms in older people *Modern Geriatrics* 2:198–212

Moen DV (1962) Observations on the effectiveness of cranberry juice in urinary infections *Wisconsin Medical Journal* 61:282–283

Moncada Iribarren I, Sáenz de Tejada I (1999) Vascular physiology of penile erection. In: Carson CC, Kirby RS, Goldstein I (eds) *Textbook of Erectile Dysfunction* Isis Medical Media, Oxford, 51–57

Montague DL, Jarow J, Broderick GA, Dmochowski R, Heaton J, Liu TF, Nchra A, Sharlip I (2004) *American Urological Association Guidelines on Pharmacologic Management of Premature Ejaculation* American Urological Association, Linthicum, MD

Moore H (1990) Caffeine. *Which?* June:314–317

Moore KN, Cody DJ, Glazener CMA (2000) Conservative management of post prostatectomy incontinence *The Cochrane Library* Issue 2, Update Software, Oxford

Moore KN, Dorey G (1999) Conservative treatment of urinary incontinence in men: a review of the literature *Physiotherapy* 85(2):77–87

Moore KN, Griffiths DJ, Hughton A (1999) A randomised controlled trial comparing pelvic muscle exercises with pelvic muscle exercises plus electrical stimulation for the treatment of post-prostatectomy urinary incontinence *British Journal of Urology* 83:57–65

Morren GL, Hallbök O, Nyström PO, Baeten CGM, Sjödahl R (2001) Audit of anal-sphincter repair *Colorectal Disease* 3:17–22

Morrison J, Birder L, Craggs M, De Groat W, Downie J, Drake M, Fowler C, Thor K (2005) Neural control. In: Abrams P, Cardozo L, Khoury S, Wein A (eds) *Incontinence*, Vol. 1, *Basics and Evaluation* Editions 21, Paris, 363–422

Moul JW (1994) For incontinence after prostatectomy, tap a diversity of treatments. *Contemporary Urology* April:78–88

Moul JW (1998) Pelvic muscle rehabilitation in males following prostatectomy. *Urologic Nursing* 18(4):296–301

Muellner SR (1960) Development of urinary control in children *Journal of the American Medical Association* 172:1256–1261

Narayan P, Konety B, Aslam K et al. (1995) Neuroanatomy of the external urethral sphincter: implications for urinary continence preservation during radical prostatectomy *Journal of Urology* 153:337–341

National Institutes of Health Consensus Development Panel on Impotence (1993) Impotence *Journal of the American Medical Association* 270:83–90

Nazareth I, Boynton P, King M (2003) Problems with sexual function in people attending London general practitioners: cross sectional study *British Medical Journal* 327:423–426

Neal DE (1997) The National Prostatectomy Audit *British Journal of Urology* 79(2):69–75

Nickel JC, Downey J, Hunter D, Clark J (2001) Prevalence of prostatitis-like symptoms in a population based study using the National Institutes of Health chronic prostatitis symptom index *Journal of Urology* 165(3):842–845

Nijman RJM, Butler R, Van Gool J, Yeung CK, Bower W, Hjalmas K (2002) Conservative management of urinary incontinence in childhood. In: Abrams P, Cardozo L, Khoury S, Wein A (eds) *Incontinence* Plymbridge Distributors Ltd, Plymouth, 515–551

Norris C (2004) *Sports Injuries* 3rd edn. Elsevier, London, 93

O'Donnell LJ, Virjee J, Heaton KW (1990) Detection of pseudodiarrhoea by simple clinical assessment of intestinal transit rate *British Medical Journal* 300(6722): 439–440

Office of Health Economics (1995) *Diseases of the Prostate* White Crescent Press, Luton

Office of Population Census and Surveys (OPCS, now called ONS) (1996) *Population Trends* No. 85, Autumn 1996. London

Opsomer RJ, Castille Y, Abi Aad AS, van Cangh PJ (1994) Urinary incontinence after radical prostatectomy: Is professional pelvic floor training necessary? *Neurourology and Urodynamics* 13(4):382–384

Palermo LM, Zimskind PD (1977) Effect of caffeine on urethral pressure *Urology* 10(4):320–324

Parekh AR, Feng MI, Kirages D et al. (2003) The role of pelvic floor exercises on post-prostatectomy incontinence *Journal of Urology* 170:130–133

Park JM, Bloom DA, McGuire EJ (1997) The guarding reflex revisited *British Journal of Urology* 80:940–945

Paterson J, Pinnock CB, Marshall, VR (1997) Pelvic floor exercises as a treatment for post-micturition dribble *British Journal of Urology* 79:892–897

Paulson DF (1991) Editorial comments *Journal of Urology* 145:515

Pettersson L, Fader M (2000) An evaluation of all-in-one incontinence pads *Nursing Times Plus* 96(6):11

Poirier P, Charpy A (1901) *Traite d'Anatomie Humaine* Masson, Paris, 197–201

Pomfret I (1993) Male incontinence *Community Outlook* March:45

Pomfret I (1996) The use of continence products. In: Norton C (ed.) *Nursing for Continence* 2nd edn. Beaconsfield Publishers, Beaconsfield, UK, 335–364

Porru D, Campus G, Caria A, Madeddu G, Cucchi A, Rovereto B, Scarpa RM, Pili P, Usai E (2001) Impact of early pelvic floor rehabilitation after transurethral resection of the prostate *Neurourology and Urodynamics* 20:53–59

Potter JM, Norton C, Cottenden A (eds) (2002) *Bowel Care in Older People: Research and Practice* Royal College of Physicians, London

Prosser EM (1938) *Manual of Massage and Movements* Faber & Faber, London, 50–52

Quain, Sharpey (1828) *Anatomy* 1st edn. London

Ralph DJ, Wylie KR (2005) Ejaculatory disorders and sexual function *British Journal of Urology International* 95:1181–1186

Resnick MI (1992) Carcinoma of the prostate. In: Resnick MI, Caldamone AA, Spirnak JP, Decker BC (eds) *Decision Making in Urology* BC Decker, Philadelphia, 114–115

Reynard J, Cannon A, Yang Q, Abrams P (1998) A novel therapy for nocturnal polyuria: a double blind randomised trial of frusemide against placebo *British Journal of Urology* 81:215–218

Robert R, Brunet C, Faure A, Lehur PA, Labat JJ, Bensignor M, Leborgne J, Barbin JY (1993) La chirurgie du nerf pudendal lors de certaines algies perineales: evolution et resultats *Chirurgie* 119:535–539

Roe B, Williams K, Palmer M (2002) Bladder training for urinary incontinence in adults *Cochrane Review* The Cochrane Library, Issue 1, Update Software, Oxford

Roehrborn CG, Van Kerrebroeck P, Nordling J (2003) Safety and efficacy of alfuzosin 10 mg once-daily in the treatment of lower urinary tract symptoms and clinical benign prostatic hyperplasia: a pooled analysis of three double-blind, placebo-controlled studies *British Journal of Urology International* 92:257–261

Rogers J (1991) Pass the cranberry juice *Nursing Times* 87(48):36–37

Rosen MP, Greenfield AJ, Walker TG, Grant P, Dubrow J, Beltmann MA, Fried LE, Goldstein I (1991) Cigarette smoking: an independent risk factor for atherosclerosis in the hypogastric-cavernous arterial bed of men with arteriogenic impotence *Journal of Urology* 145(4):759–763

Rosen RC (2000) Prevalence and risk factors of sexual dysfunction in men and women *Current Psychiatry* Rep 2:189–195

Rosser BR, Short BJ, Thurmes PJ, Coleman E (1998) Anodyspareunia, the unacknowledged sexual dysfunction: a validation study of painful receptive anal intercourse and its psychosexual concomitants in homosexual men *Journal of Sex and Marital Therapy* 24(4):281–292

Rowland D (2003) The treatment of premature ejaculation: selecting outcomes to determine efficacy *International Society for Sexual and Impotence Research Newsbulletin* 10:26–28

Rowland D et al. (2004) Self-reported premature ejaculation and aspects of sexual functioning and satisfaction *Journal of Sexual Medicine* 1:225–232

Rudy DC, Woodside JR, Crawford ED (1984) Urodynamic evaluation of incontinence in patients undergoing modified Campbell radical retro pubic prostatectomy: a prospective study *Journal of Urology* 132:708–712

Sackett DL (1986) How are we to determine whether dietary interventions do more good than harm to hypertensive patients? *Canadian Journal of Physiology and Pharmacology* 64(6):781–783

Salmons S, Henriksonn J (1981) The adaptive response of skeletal muscle to increased use *Muscle and Nerve* 4:94–105

Sant GR, Long JP (1994) Benign prostatic hyperplasia. In: Sant GR (ed.) *Pathophysiologic Principles of Urology* Blackwell Scientific Publications, London, 123–154

Sapsford RR, Hodges PW, Richardson CA et al. (2001) Co-activation of the abdominal and pelvic floor muscles during voluntary exercise *Neurourology and Urodynamics* 20:31–42

Schurch B, Reitz A (2004) Botulinum toxin in urology *Urologe A* 43(11):1410–1415

Schuster MM (1990) Rectal pain *Current Therapy for Gastroenterologic Liver Disease* 3:378–379

Shafik A, El-Sibai O (2000) The anocavernosal erectile dysfunction syndrome: II, Anal fissure and erectile dysfunction *International Journal of Impotence Research* 12:279–283

Shelly B, Knight S, King P et al. (2002) Assessment of pelvic pain. In: Laycock J, Haslam J (eds) *Therapeutic Management of Incontinence and Pelvic Pain* Springer-Verlag, Berlin, 171–176

Simons DG, Travell JG, Simon LS (1999) *Myofascial Pain and Dysfunction. The Trigger Point Manual* 2nd edn. Williams & Wilkins, Baltimore, MD, Vol. 1

Simpson RJ, Fisher W, Lee AJ, Russell EBAW, Garraway M (1996) Benign prostatic hyperplasia in an unselected community-based population: a survey of urinary symptoms, bothersomeness and prostatic enlargement *British Journal of Urology* 77:186–191

Siroky MB (1996) Electromyography of the perineal floor *Urologic Clinics of North America* 23(2):299–307

Smith M (1997) Trickle of information *Nursing Times Suppl.* 93:5

Sommer F, Raible A, Bondarenko B, Caspers HP, Esders K, Bartsch G, Schoenenberger A, Engelmann U (2002) A conservative treatment option of curing venous leakage in impotent men *European Urology Supplement* (Abstract) 1(1):153

Sotiropoulos A, Yeaw S, Lattimer JK (1976) Management of urinary incontinence with electronic stimulation: observations and results *Journal of Urology* 116:747–750

Stainbrook E (1948) The use of electricity in psychiatric treatment during the nineteenth century *Bulletin History Medicine* 22:156–177

Stanford JL, Feng Z, Hamilton AS et al. (2000) Urinary and sexual function after radical prostatectomy for clinically localized prostate cancer: the Prostate Cancer Outcomes Study *Journal of American Medical Association* 283(3):354–360

Steege JF (1998) Scope of the problem. In: Steege JF, Metzger DA, Levy BA (eds) *Chronic Pelvic Pain: An Integrated Approach* W.B. Saunders, Philadelphia, 1–4

Steers WD (1992) Physiology of the urinary bladder. In: Walsh PC, Retik AB, Stamey TA, Vaughan JR (eds) *Campbell's Urology* W.B. Saunders, Philadelphia, 142–178

Stephenson TP, Farrar DJ (1977) Urodynamic study of 15 patients with postmicturition dribble *Urology* 9(4):404–406

Stief CG, Weller E, Noack T, Djamilian, MH, Meschi M, Truss M, Jonas U (1996) Functional electromyostimulation of the penile corpus cavernosum (FEMCC). Initial results of a new therapeutic option of erectile dysfunction *Urologe A* 35(4):321–325

Strasser H, Steinlechner M, Bartsch G (1997) Morphometric analysis of the rhabdo-sphincter of the male urethra *Journal of Urology* 157(Suppl. 4):177

Sueppel C, Kreder K, See W (2001) Improved continence outcomes with preoperative pelvic floor muscle strengthening exercises *Urologic Nursing* 21(3):201–210

Thiele GH (1937) Coccygodynia and pain in the superior gluteal region *Journal of American Medical Association* 109:1271–1274

Thomas TM, Plymat KR, Blannin J, Meade TW (1980) Prevalence of urinary incontinence *British Medical Journal* 281(6250):1243–1245

Torrens M (1987) Human physiology. In: Torrens M, Morrison JFB (eds) *Physiology of the Lower Urinary Tract* Springer-Verlag, London, 33–350

Trueman P, Hood SC, Nayak USL, Mrazek MF (1999) Prevalence of lower urinary tract symptoms and self-reported diagnosed 'benign prostatic hyperplasia', and their effect on quality of life in a community-based survey of men in the UK *British Journal of Urology International* 83:410–415

Upledger J (2005) CranioSacral Therapy Fact Sheet. www.upledger.com

Van Driel MF, Van de Wiel HBM, Mensink HJA (1994) Some mythological, religious and cultural aspects of impotence before the present modern era. *International Journal of Impotence Research* 6:163–169

Van Kampen M, De Weerdt W, Van Poppel H, De Ridder D, Feys H, Baert L (2000) The effect of physiotherapy on the duration and the degree of incontinence after radical prostatectomy: a randomised controlled trial *The Lancet* 355(9198):98–102

Van Kampen M, De Weerdt W, Claes H, Feys H, De Maeyer M, Van Poppel H (2003) Treatment of erectile dysfunction by perineal exercises, electromyographic biofeedback and electrical stimulation *Physical Therapy* 83(6):536–543

Van Kerrebroeck P, Weiss J (1999) Standardization and terminology of nocturia. *British Journal of Urology International* 84(Suppl. 1):1–4

Vereecken RL, Verduyn H (1970) The electrical activity of the paraurethral and perineal muscles in normal and pathological conditions *British Journal of Urology* 42:457–463

Vereecken RL, Wouters M (1988) Discrepancies between clinical and urodynamic findings: Which are true? *Urology International* 43:282

Vestey SB, Hinchcliffe A (1998) The frequency/volume (F/V) chart: don't be without one! *British Journal of Urology* 81(Suppl. 4):21

Vidler U (1964) *Physiotherapy as a Career.* Batson Ltd, London, 18–19

Wagg A, Malone-Lee J (1999) Problems in elderly people. In: Wagg A, Malone-Lee J (eds) *Bladder Problems* Martin Dunitz, London, 44–51

Wagner TH, Patrick DL, McKenna SP, Froese PS (1996) Cross-cultural development of a quality of life measure for men with erection difficulties *Quality of Life Research* 5:443–449

Waldinger MD, Hengeveld MW, Zwinderman AH, Olivier, B (1998) An empirical operationalization study of DSM-IV diagnostic criteria for premature ejaculation *International Journal of Psychiatric Practice* 2:287

Wasserman IF (1964) Puborectalis syndrome *Diseases of Colon and Rectum* 7:87–98

Wein AW (1997) Pharmacologic options for the overactive bladder *Urology* 51(Suppl. 2A):43–47

Weisberg HF (1982) *Water, Electrolyte and Acid-base Balance* 2nd edn. Williams & Wilkins, Baltimore

Wells TJ (1988) Additional treatments for urinary incontinence *Topics in Geriatric Rehabilitation* 3(2):48–57

Wesselmann U, Burnett AL, Heinberg LJ (1997) The urogenital and rectal pain syndromes *Pain* 73:269–294

Wheelahan J, Scott NA, Cartmill R, Marshall V, Morton RP, Nacey J, Maddern GJ (The ASERNIP-S review group) (2000) Minimally invasive non-laser thermal techniques for prostatectomy: a systematic review *British Journal of Urology International* 86:977–988

Wilson PD, Glazener C, McGee M et al. (2002) Randomised controlled trial of conservative management of postnatal urinary and faecal incontinence: long-term follow-up study *Neurourology and Urodynamics* 21:370

Wilt TJ, Ishani A, Stark G, MacDonald R, Lau J, Mulrow C (1998) Saw palmetto extracts for treatment of benign prostatic hyperplasia: a systematic review *Journal of the American Medical Association* 280(18):1604–1609

Wisinski C, Rolf-Carbaugh L, Bangs KA (2001) Physical therapy for urinary incontinence utilizing rectal weights following radical prostatectomy *Journal of the Section on Women's Health* 25(4):9–11

World Health Organization (1978) Definition of Health. World Health Organization, Geneva

World Health Organization (1992) International statistical classification of diseases and related health problems. 1989 Revision. World Health Organization, Geneva

Wyndaele JJ, Van Eetvelde B (1996) Reproducibility of digital testing of the pelvic floor muscles in men *Archives of Physical Medicine and Rehabilitation* 77(11):1179–1181

Xin ZC, Choi YD, Rha KH, Choi HK (1997) Somatosensory evoked potentials in patients with primary premature ejaculation *Journal of Urology* 158(2):451–455

Xin ZC, Chung WS, Choi YD et al. (1996) Penile sensitivity in patients with primary premature ejaculation *Journal of Urology* 156(3):979–981

Zermann DH, Ishigooka M, Doggweiler-Wiygul R et al. (2001) The male chronic pelvic pain syndrome *World Journal of Urology* 19(3):173–179

Index